HYPNOSIS
FOR SUCCESSFUL
MINDS

A Practical Guide to Rapid Results
and Deep Inner Work

CHERRY FARROW

HYPNOSIS
FOR SUCCESSFUL
MINDS

A Practical Guide to Rapid Results
and Deep Inner Work

First Edition 2026 v1.2

Hypnosis For Successful Minds

A Practical Guide to Rapid Results and Deep Inner Work

ASIN: B0GSQ2CX5C (Amazon Kindle)
eBook ISBN: 978-1-923223-82-0
Amazon Paperback ISBN: 978-1-923223-81-3
Amazon Hardcover ISBN: 978-1-923223-84-4
IngramSpark Paperback ISBN: 978-1-923223-83-7
IngramSpark Hardcover ISBN: 978-1-923223-85-1

Table of Contents

Acknowledgements

This book would not have been possible without the incredible support, love and belief of so many people — each of whom has played a role in bringing *Hypnosis for Successful Minds* to life.

To my clients — you are the reason I do this work. Thank you for trusting me to walk beside you as you healed, transformed and found your power. Your journeys inspired every chapter.

To my students and graduates — thank you for your courage, your commitment and your hunger to help others. Watching you step into mastery continues to be one of the greatest privileges of my life.

To the team at Successful Minds Institute — your dedication, care and brilliance behind the scenes allow this mission to reach hearts and minds across the globe.

To my family — thank you for being the roots beneath everything I do. Your love is my home.

And to those who walk the path of transformation, healing and contribution — thank you. This book is for you.

Dedication

For the seekers, the healers, the cycle-breakers and the ones who have always known there is more.

More to who we are. More to what we're capable of. More to the mind's ability to heal, evolve and create lasting change.

You're the ones who choose growth over comfort — the ones who believe transformation is possible — and that it starts within.

You are part of a new wave of changemakers — those who blend science with soul, structure with intuition and purpose with compassion.

This book is for you. For the difference you're here to make. For the lives you'll touch. For the future you'll help shape.

With every person you support, you help build a global community of MindFit™ individuals — clear, confident and aligned with something greater than themselves.

You were made for this. And now, it's time.

About the Author

Cherry Farrow is a Master Trainer of Neuro-Linguistic Programming and Hypnosis, creator of The Release System™, the Quantum Healing Paradigm™ and founder of *Successful Minds Institute*, an internationally recognised training organisation dedicated to unlocking human potential and cultivating a global community of MindFit™ individuals.

With over two decades of experience helping thousands of students and clients around the world, Cherry is known for her warm, empowering teaching style and ability to make the most complex transformational tools easy to understand, elegant to use and profoundly effective.

Her signature approach blends science, soul and deep therapeutic skill. She has trained individuals from all walks of life — coaches, therapists, doctors, psychologists, military personnel, teachers, executives and parents — to become confident communicators and ethical change-makers through a deep understanding of the Unconscious Mind.

At the heart of Cherry's work is a simple belief: when people truly understand how their mind works, lasting healing, growth and success become natural outcomes.

Hypnosis for Successful Minds is her practical gift to the next generation of hypnotherapists — those ready to trust the process, master the craft and make a meaningful, lasting difference.

Foreword

Cherry Farrow has masterfully written an excellent book for both the newbie and seasoned professional alike.

As a practitioner in all aspects of the Hypnotic arts for over 40 years, I believe Cherry has brought something interesting to your conscious mind that you can download into your unconscious (other than conscious) mind. It's an excellent book that fills many gaps in this profession that every practitioner and curiosity seeker would be wise to have on their bookshelf.

Over the years, I have reviewed countless books from colleagues who wanted my input on their material. However, this is the first time I have actually been excited enough to respond. The reason is that Cherry really gets it, loves it, applies it, and is now sharing it.

Everything from basic hypnosis to advanced therapeutic interventions. It's all here. Just absorb the information as if you are bathing in a warm bath with jets of water gently massaging your body into relaxation.

Reading through her book a few times now, it felt like time distortion, going back to hypnosis school, with fantastic upgrades, that 3 months from now you'll be able to look back on having found this book, read it and applying the principles with a smile on your face.

To recap: this book is a must-read for anyone serious about the art and science of Hypnosis & Hypnotherapy as it opens the door to so many possibilities you may have not yet considered.

I'm just wondering if you will enjoy this as much as I have and how you will employ these techniques to refine your present work, will you not?

Keep on Trancin'

Don Spencer
www.SleepNow.com

(About the Author of the Foreword)

Don Spencer, known internationally as *'Spencer the World's Fastest Hypnotist'*, is a renowned stage hypnotist, clinical hypnotherapist, and trainer who has spent more than four decades demonstrating the extraordinary potential of the human mind.

In addition to his therapeutic and training work, Spencer became known for pioneering large-scale hypnosis entertainment and innovation, including presenting what has been described as the world's first holographic hypnosis performance in Australia. Through his performances, teachings, and mentorship, Don Spencer has helped bring hypnosis to audiences around the world while inspiring a new generation of practitioners to explore the remarkable power of the unconscious mind.

Chapter 1:

Introduction – The Mind/Body Connection

Welcome to the transformative world of hypnosis, where you'll first uncover the techniques that have shaped the field and then master them to create profound change in yourself and others. Throughout this book, we'll explore a wide range of approaches — from the indirect, permissive style of Milton Erickson to the more direct, authoritative methods of pioneers like George Estabrooks. No matter the approach, the true power of hypnosis lies in the relationship you create with the **Unconscious Mind**— both your own and your client's.

The magic and benefits of hypnosis emerge from the trance state. In the pages ahead, you'll learn to harness the ability to produce and work with deep trance phenomena. Your capacity to move from your current state into a deep trance relies heavily on the rapport you develop with your Unconscious Mind. We'll explore how to strengthen that connection and work with it at deeper levels — not only to facilitate your personal growth but also to empower every client you work with.

The Connection Between the Unconscious Mind and the Body

The gateway to success in hypnosis is through the Unconscious Mind. This part of you is far more than a repository of untapped thoughts or memories — it is also the manager of your body's sensations and functions. Consider this: before reading this sentence, were you consciously aware of the pressure of your feet on the floor or the sensation of your back against the chair? Likely not. Your Unconscious Mind is constantly processing sensations and stimuli, yet you remain unaware of most of them.

More than just managing sensations, your Unconscious Mind ensures that vital functions, like your heartbeat, blood circulation, digestion and lymphatic system continue seamlessly – it even makes your eyes blink – all without requiring your conscious attention. It is awe-inspiring to realise that your Unconscious Mind orchestrates these complex processes with perfect precision.

One of the foundational concepts you'll explore here is the understanding that your Unconscious Mind is in constant communication with every cell in your body.

Early skeptics dismissed hypnosis as something that existed 'only in the mind'. However advances in neuroscience, psychoneuroimmunology, and epigenetics have changed that view entirely. Researchers such as Candace Pert and Ernest Rossi have demonstrated that thoughts, emotions, and mental states are closely linked with neurochemical signals that influence immune function, hormonal activity, and cellular processes throughout the body. In other words, the language of the mind is constantly shaping the experience of the body.

This revelation highlights a profound truth: the techniques you're about to learn not only create shifts in the mind but they also ripple through the body, fostering healing, growth and transformation. As you continue this journey, you'll deepen your understanding of this connection and discover how to use it to bring about remarkable results for yourself and those you serve.

The Mind/Body Connection in Action

Information flows through the body as electrical impulses travelling along nerve cells (or neurons). Between each pair of neurons is a small gap, called a synapse, which these impulses must cross to continue their journey. The fascinating task of bridging these gaps is carried out by neurotransmitters — specialised chemicals that conduct electrical impulses across synapses.

When neurotransmitters were first discovered, scientists believed they existed only in the brain. However, further research revealed that neurotransmitters connect all neurons in the body, creating an intricate network of 'electrical circuits'. Advances in quantum physics and quantum biology have since expanded our understanding, showing that neurotransmitters bathe every single cell in the human body. This groundbreaking insight has become the cornerstone of understanding the mind/body connection.

In this model of hypnosis, it's recognised that your Unconscious Mind not only manages sensations, movements and body functions — it also sends information that impacts billions of cells in your body. These messages, shaped by your unconscious beliefs, influence your state of health or dis-ease.

Modern research in psychoneuroimmunology suggests that the immune system is continuously responding to signals generated by our thoughts, emotions and perceptions. In other words, your immune system is constantly listening to your internal dialogue and adjusting its responses accordingly.

But it's not just the words you say to yourself. From the perspective of hypnosis and Neuro-Linguistic Programming (NLP), your immune system also responds to the images you hold in your mind, the sounds you pay attention to, the feelings you experience and the concepts you focus on. Thanks to the conductivity of neurotransmitters surrounding all your cells, the activity of your Unconscious Mind continuously affects your physical well-being.

While there are many aspects of our lives we consciously manage, the optimal operation and health of the body is orchestrated by the Unconscious Mind. Hypnosis offers us the ability to access this unconscious realm, creating a direct pathway to tap into the power of the mind/body connection.

Through the methods shared in this book – developed over years of clinical work and teaching – you'll discover how to engage this connection intentionally. This is the gateway to manifesting incredible outcomes in health, personal transformation and overall well-being.

The Unreality of Reality

As we explore the fascinating workings of the Unconscious Mind, one question arises time and again: What is real? This question belongs solely to the Conscious Mind, as the Unconscious Mind does not operate within the boundaries of what we call 'reality'. At the level of the Unconscious Mind, there is no distinction between what is 'real' and what is not.

But let's push this further: Is the Unconscious Mind real?

The word 'real' implies having substance, something tangible and measurable. By that definition, the Unconscious Mind itself is not 'real'. This leads us to another question: What is 'real' about hypnosis and the connection between the mind and body?

The answer lies in the remarkable bridge that connects the mind and body. This bridge not only links the physical with the mental but also allows us to move between the realms of the 'real' and the 'unreal'. If we accept that the 'real' is confined to the physical, then we must consider the 'unreality' of the mind — and therein lies the key to transformation.

The Perspective of the Shaman

The wisdom of the Shaman teaches us that the world around us is not truly real. When this understanding resonates, you'll have embraced the 'unreality' of what we perceive as reality — a state of heightened awareness. This realisation is not new. Zen Buddhists spend decades meditating on paradoxical koans, striving to grasp that all reality begins with the perception and intention of the mind.

For practitioners of hypnosis, this awareness is a game-changer. Understanding the 'unreality of reality' helps us see the body as just another expression of the mind. The body, like the rest of reality, is malleable and can transform rapidly, even instantly. With this awareness, you can harness the power to support your own healing and guide others to do the same, addressing anything from high blood pressure to metabolic imbalances to disease.

A Remarkable Case: The Power of the Mind

One of the most intriguing cases I was told about early in my training came from a mentor deeply immersed in mind–body work and hypnosis. It involved a woman who experienced herself through multiple personality states, each with its own distinct patterns of perception, emotion and physiology.

In one state, she experienced herself as diabetic. In another, she did not.

What made this case so compelling was not the label, but the observable shift that occurred when she moved from one personality state to another. When she was operating from the personality that identified as diabetic, her body behaved accordingly. Yet when she transitioned into a different personality — one that held no identity or expectation of diabetes — her physiology responded in a dramatically different way.

The change occurred almost immediately, far more rapidly than would be expected through ordinary physical processes alone.

This case raises profound questions — questions that sit at the very heart of hypnosis and the mind/body connection:

What is the true cause of illness or wellness? What is real — the body, the mind, or the beliefs that organise both?

From the perspective of hypnosis, the answer points us toward the extraordinary influence of the Unconscious Mind. It suggests that the body is not merely a fixed biological machine, but a dynamic system continually responding to unconscious identity, expectation and internal communication.

This understanding does not require us to abandon science — it invites us to expand it.

When the Unconscious Mind organises reality differently, the body responds accordingly. Hypnosis gives us a bridge into that organising principle, allowing us to work at the level where perception, belief and physiology meet.

It is at this level — beyond logic, beyond conscious effort — that profound transformation becomes possible.

Metaphysically Speaking: The Unity of the Mind

At its core, the mind is one, a seamless and interconnected entity. However, since most people don't experience it that way, the distinction between the Conscious Mind and the Unconscious Mind becomes a valuable tool. While some behaviourists may argue against the existence of an Unconscious Mind, this division allows us to more clearly understand how our minds operate and influence our lives.

Why Learn Hypnosis?

The value of learning hypnosis — and experiencing trance — lies in unlocking profound power: the power to heal your own body and guide others to do the same; the power to learn effortlessly and deeply; and the power to create lasting changes in your life and the lives of others.

Imagine being able to produce hypnotic phenomena in yourself, such as arm catalepsy (rigidity), deep muscle relaxation, or even full-body catalepsy. If you can achieve that, you can also guide your Unconscious Mind to initiate healing.

Some examples of the healing power include:

- Pain relief: If you experience severe muscle tension in your back, imagine the relief of simply sitting down, entering trance and communicating directly with your *Unconscious Mind: Dear Unconscious Mind, go ahead and release the tension in the muscles in my back and allow it to heal safely and healthily.* With clear communication and rapport, this becomes entirely possible.

- Healing visualisation: If you can hallucinate a tennis ball (yes you will learn how), you can just as easily visualise a beam of golden light moving through your body and imagine it as a powerful cleansing wave. This wave flows gently but relentlessly, dissolving any dis-eased cells, toxins or blockages in its path. Like sunlight burning away the morning mist, this healing light restores balance and health to every part of your body it touches.

Today, there is a groundswell of support for the healing potential of hypnosis within the traditional medical community. Increasingly, allopathic medicine recognises hypnosis as a complementary tool for physical and emotional well-being.

Opening New Doors to Learning

The Unconscious Mind is also a gateway to accelerated learning.

If you want to absorb new information easily, simply say, *Dear Unconscious Mind, let's learn this and organise it so it is easy to remember, easy to recall and easy to utilise.* Trust in its support.

If you're preparing for an important presentation, communicate with your Unconscious Mind, saying, "Dear Unconscious Mind, let's organise this presentation to be engaging and to flow easily and effortlessly."

Your mind is your greatest ally when you give it clear direction.

Creating Real Change in Your Life

In trance, you access the real power to:

- heal what needs to be healed

- preserve valuable learnings from the past

- forge new neurological connections to manifest your dreams.

One technique you'll be introduced to is The Release System™, which I developed and teach to hundreds of students each year, enabling them to release negative emotions, limiting beliefs and blocks while empowering them to create a compelling and purposeful future.

As Milton Erickson once said: *Patients are patients because they are out of rapport with their own Unconscious.*

People often lose rapport with their Unconscious Minds due to years of outside programming — expectations, societal conditioning and emotional baggage. Hypnosis reconnects people to their inner selves, giving them the resources to take control of their lives and their destiny.

Becoming Superb Hypnotherapists and Skilled Subjects

Throughout this journey, we'll explore hypnosis for two key purposes:

1. To become exceptional hypnotherapists — guiding clients to experience the rich benefits of trance, healing and transformation.

2. To become proficient hypnotic subjects — learning to access those same benefits ourselves by entering deep, healing and transformational trance states.

Whether your goal is to heal, to learn, or to create profound change, hypnosis is the bridge that allows you to harness the power of your Unconscious Mind. When you are in rapport with your Unconscious, you are in alignment with your true potential—and from there, anything becomes possible.

Chapter 2:

A Brief History of Hypnosis

Before exploring how hypnosis works, let's delve into its fascinating history. Understanding the journey of hypnosis will deepen your appreciation for this powerful art and its techniques.

Early Foundations

The practice of hypnosis can be traced back thousands of years. Ancient Sanskrit writings from India describe healing trances and temples dedicated to therapeutic rituals. Similarly, Egyptian papyrus scrolls detail the use of sleeping temples and trance inductions for healing purposes. These early practices reveal that hypnosis, in its essence, has been intertwined with human healing for centuries.

The Renaissance and Magnetism

In the 1500s, Paracelsus, a Swiss physician, pioneered the use of magnets in healing. He would pass a magnet or lodestone over a person's body to initiate recovery. This method proved effective for curing various diseases.

In the 1600s, Valentine Greatrakes, an Irish healer nicknamed 'The Great Irish Stroker', became famous for using his hands and in some accounts magnets to massage ailments out of the body.

Franz Anton Mesmer and Animal Magnetism

The 1700s marked a turning point with the methods of Franz Anton Mesmer, a Viennese doctor who built upon the work of his teacher, Maximilian

Hell. Mesmer initially used magnets to stop bleeding during medical procedures. Once, lacking a magnet, he used another object — and it worked. This led Mesmer to conclude that it wasn't the object itself, but the magnetic energy emanating from the patient. He termed this *Animal Magnetism*.

Mesmer's theories became immensely popular, especially among the French aristocracy. However, controversy arose when the medical establishment questioned his methods. Upon Mesmer's request, King Louis XVI appointed a Board of Inquiry, consisting of notable figures, including chemist Antoine Lavoisier, inventor Benjamin Franklin, and physician Dr Guillotin. The Board concluded that the observed effects were due to imagination rather than a measurable physical force. While this discredited Mesmer's Animal Magnetism as a physical theory, it unintentionally highlighted the power of suggestion - a cornerstone of modern hypnosis.

Evolution of Hypnotic States

Mesmer's successor, Marquis de Puységur, observed that deep trances resembled a sleepwalking state, which he called *somnambulism*. This term is still used to describe the deepest states of hypnosis. By the early 1800s, figures like Dr John Elliotson integrated mesmerism into their medical practices in London, often facing resistance from the traditional medical community.

The Birth of Hypnosis

In 1841, surgeon James Braid revolutionised the field after observing mesmerist Charles Lafontaine demonstrate 'animal magnetism' in Manchester. Braid noticed the significance of eye fixation in inducing a trance. He introduced the term *hypnotism* (from his earlier neuro-hypnology), and the field later adopted the term *hypnosis*. Braid theorised that hypnosis was not due to magnetic energy but the result of suggestion and focused attention. In his seminal book *Neurypnology* (1843), he emphasised that fixation on a single idea or point triggers hypnosis. Though he later proposed the term *monoideaism*, hypnosis remained the accepted term.

Around the same time, James Esdaile, a British doctor in India, used mesmerism for pain control during surgeries, performing between 300-500 operations without anesthetics. His success highlighted hypnosis's potential in medicine, although skepticism and the advent of chloroform overshadowed his contributions.

Hypnosis and the Nancy School

By 1864, Ambroise Liébault established a therapeutic system using hypnosis in Nancy, France, marking a major shift in the understanding of hypnotic phenomena. Unlike earlier mesmerists, Liébault viewed hypnosis not as a magnetic or mysterious force, but as a natural psychological state shaped by suggestion.

His collaboration with neurologist Hippolyte Bernheim led to the development of what became known as the Nancy School of Hypnosis. Together, they demonstrated that suggestion alone, whether in a light trance or even in the waking state, could influence perception, sensation, and physiological responses. They documented successful outcomes in conditions such as pain syndromes, functional disorders, and psychosomatic illnesses, including sciatica.

More importantly, the Nancy School established that hypnosis operates along a continuum, rather than as a distinct or pathological state. This understanding reframed hypnosis as an extension of everyday psychological processes such as attention, imagination, and belief. Their work profoundly influenced the emerging fields of psychotherapy and psychosomatic medicine, and attracted many students, including a young Sigmund Freud, who initially adopted their methods before later developing psychoanalysis.

The Nancy School's emphasis on suggestion as the primary mechanism of change laid the foundation for modern clinical hypnosis, cognitive-behavioural approaches, and later developments in Ericksonian hypnosis and NLP.

Freud and Hypnosis

Freud initially incorporated hypnosis into his practice after studying at the Nancy School, but later abandoned it. Publicly, he cited its unpredictability and the intensity of emotional transference as reasons for moving away from hypnosis. Some historians have also speculated that Freud's personal health issues and substance use may have made hypnotic work more challenging for him. He subsequently developed psychoanalysis, which dominated European psychology and temporarily eclipsed hypnosis.

Modern Developments

In 1890, psychologist William James published *The Principles of Psychology*, a seminal work that continues to influence hypnosis and NLP practitioners today. James explored attention, habit, consciousness, and voluntary control, offering insights that align closely with hypnotic phenomena. During this period, behaviourism also emerged as a counterpoint to Freudian psychoanalysis, shifting psychology's focus toward observable stimulus–response patterns.

Around the same time, important groundwork for conditioning was laid by Edwin B. Twitmyer, who in 1902 observed conditioned reflexes in humans through knee-jerk response experiments, later presenting his findings in 1904. These early observations closely paralleled and were later expanded upon by Ivan Pavlov, whose research on conditioned reflexes in dogs became widely recognised. Together, these developments helped establish a scientific understanding of stimulus and response — principles that underpin suggestion, learning, and hypnotic responsiveness.

Hypnosis in the 20th Century

In 1933, Clark Hull published *Hypnosis and Suggestibility*, a groundbreaking psychological study. Hull proposed the principle that 'any procedure that assumes a trance can facilitate trance' highlighting the flexibility of hypnotic induction methods. Techniques like progressive relaxation and creative visualisation are rooted in this concept.

Hull's work influenced Milton H. Erickson, a pioneering hypnotherapist whose indirect, permissive style transformed hypnosis into a modern therapeutic art. Erickson's profound insights and innovative techniques feature prominently in this book. Dave Elman also played a significant role in contemporary hypnosis, particularly in medical and clinical applications. His methods emphasised rapid inductions and practical approaches to achieve deep states of trance quickly and reliably. Elman's techniques, including the famous Elman Induction, are highly effective in therapeutic and clinical settings and will be explored in depth through our Master Practitioner Hypnosis Training and Quantum Healing Paradigm™ Training, which is part of the Clinical Diploma of Hypnotherapy & NLP.

Another notable figure, George Estabrooks, further advanced the applications of hypnosis, blending clinical practice with experimental research.

The Contributions of André Weitzenhoffer and LeCron

André Weitzenhoffer, co-author with Ernest Hilgard, of the influential book *Hypnotic Susceptibility*, made significant contributions to the scientific study of hypnosis. His work provided a deeper understanding of suggestibility and the mechanisms underlying trance.

Leslie M. LeCron, another pioneering figure, introduced the concept of ideomotor signalling — a powerful tool for communicating directly with the unconscious mind. Using a pendulum or finger movements, ideomotor responses allow clients to answer questions or access insights without conscious interference. This technique, which will be covered in this training, is invaluable for uncovering root causes of issues and facilitating profound change.

Direct vs Indirect and Authoritarian vs Permissive Approaches

Hypnosis techniques can vary widely, often categorised as direct or indirect and authoritarian or permissive.

Direct hypnosis involves explicit suggestions like 'You will now relax', while indirect hypnosis, championed by Milton Erickson, uses stories, metaphors and subtle language patterns to guide the subject into trance.

Similarly, an authoritarian approach relies on commanding language, assuming a position of control, whereas a permissive approach gently invites the subject to explore their own experience. Both methods have their place in modern hypnosis, depending on the client's needs and preferences. This book, which complements our training, will provide you with tools to apply both styles effectively, ensuring versatility in your practice.

The Legacy of Hypnosis

This historical journey is not merely academic. Each era reflects a shift in how we understand the mind, suggestion, and change, principles that directly inform the techniques you will learn and apply throughout this book.

From ancient healing temples to modern therapeutic methods, hypnosis has evolved through centuries of innovation, skepticism and rediscovery. Each contribution — from Mesmer's Animal Magnetism to Erickson's conversational techniques — has enriched this powerful discipline. By understanding its history, we gain deeper insights into the immense potential of hypnosis for healing, transformation and personal growth.

As hypnosis evolved, so too did the responsibility of the practitioner, highlighting the importance of ethics, consent, and clinical skill in working with the unconscious mind.

Chapter 3:

Understanding the Conscious and Unconscious Mind in Hypnosis

The Dance Between Logic and Imagination

Before you learn how to guide someone into trance; before you give powerful suggestions; and before you even begin to help someone change … you need to understand who you're actually talking to when you speak in hypnosis.

Why?

In hypnosis, we're not really speaking to the logical, analytical conscious mind. We're speaking directly to the deeper, wiser, more powerful part … the Unconscious Mind.

Let's explore the difference.

The Conscious Mind: The Flashlight of Awareness

You can think of the Conscious Mind like a flashlight. It shines a narrow beam of focus on just one thing at a time.

It's the part of you that:

- does the shopping list

- analyses problems

- worries about the future

- thinks in words and logic

- follows step-by-step instructions.

The Conscious Mind is:

- analytical (it breaks things down and evaluates them)

- sequential (it processes one thing at a time)

- cognitive (it does your thinking and reasoning)

- logical (it needs reasons, evidence and explanation)

- deliberate (it works with conscious willpower and choice).

The Conscious Mind also has limited focus (it can only hold seven-plus-or-minus-two bits of information at once). It directs your outcomes and controls your thinking (though, not always your feelings), and it is most active when you're awake and alert.

As powerful as it sounds, however, the Conscious Mind is actually very limited. It's like the tip of the iceberg — you can see it, but there's so much more underneath.

The Unconscious Mind: The Floodlight of Possibility

Now picture the Unconscious Mind as a floodlight. It doesn't focus on just one thing; it picks up everything at once, all the time.

This is the part of you that:

- keeps your heart beating

- stores all your memories

- dreams at night

- feels your gut instincts

- runs your habits automatically.

The Unconscious Mind is:

- unlimited (it processes millions of bits of data per second)

- expansive (it connects to every cell in your body)

- active (it never turns off, even when you're sleeping and dreaming)

- simultaneous (it can do many things at once)

- feeling (it communicates through sensations, emotions and images)

- intuitive (it notices patterns and makes leaps in understanding).

The Unconscious Mind is also responsible for your involuntary movements, such as breathing and digestion. And it knows the solutions to problems, even when the Conscious Mind doesn't.

The Unconscious Mind is your inner genius. It's your internal guidance system, and the true target of all hypnotic work.

A Simple Example to Remember It

Let's play for a moment. Imagine I tell you to "Jump out of your chair and fly to the moon."

Your Conscious Mind immediately says, "That's impossible. I can't do that."

Instead, let me say, "Close your eyes and imagine flying out of your chair, soaring past the stars and circling the moon."

Your Unconscious Mind may say, "Sure!"

Suddenly, you're floating effortlessly through space.

The Conscious Mind limits. The Unconscious Mind expands.

This is the beauty of hypnosis — we bypass the limitations of logic and speak directly to the part of the mind that believes in miracles and makes change possible.

Why Does This Matter in Hypnosis?

People may say:

- "I want to stop smoking, but I just can't."

- "I know I'm safe, but I still feel anxious."

- "I want confidence, but I freeze in front of people."

These are not conscious problems. They are unconscious patterns. Trying to fix them with conscious willpower alone is like trying to dig a well with a spoon.

Instead, we should go straight to the Unconscious Mind — the part that already knows what needs to change and how.

Bypassing the Critical Faculty

Between the Conscious and Unconscious Mind is something we call the Critical Faculty.

Think of it like a bouncer at the door of a VIP club. It decides what gets through to your unconscious and what doesn't.

If a suggestion makes sense and fits your beliefs, the bouncer lets it in.

If it sounds silly, threatening, or unfamiliar, the bouncer keeps it out.

Hypnosis, however, is like a VIP pass. It helps you gently bypass that critical gatekeeper so new ideas, helpful suggestions and positive changes can get in and start working.

How the Critical Faculty Forms

If you've ever wondered why children can believe in magic, monsters and the absolute power of a Band-Aid — without hesitation — you're beginning to understand something powerful about the mind.

Children aren't born with the ability to question everything. In fact, they come into the world like open sponges — soaking up every idea, belief and suggestion without filtering them or resisting.

That filtering mechanism — the part of the mind that begins to say, "Wait a minute … is that really true?" —doesn't exist in the early years. This mental gatekeeper — the Critical Faculty — plays a major role in hypnosis.

Understanding how and when the Critical Faculty forms helps you appreciate why hypnosis works so effectively — especially when we bypass this filter and speak directly to the Unconscious Mind.

Let's look at what developmental psychology, hypnosis research and Neuro-Linguistic Programming (NLP) have shown us about this mysterious part of the mind.

Jean Piaget's Stages of Cognitive Development

Piaget, a leading developmental psychologist, identified that children move from the preoperational stage (2–7 years) into the concrete operational stage (7–11 years). During this transition, children:

- begin to think logically about concrete events

- gain the ability to understand perspectives and question ideas.

This marks the beginning of internal critical evaluation, which is a foundation of the Critical Faculty.

Hypnosis and Suggestibility Research

Studies in hypnotherapy and suggestibility show that children under the age of seven are naturally in a highly suggestible state. They tend to accept new ideas without question. From around the age of seven, and up to eleven, children are less susceptible to suggestion as they start applying logic, doubt and skepticism. This indicates that the Critical Faculty is taking shape.

Educational Psychology Observations

Teachers and educators often notice a developmental shift with younger children readily believing in Santa Claus, the Tooth Fairy and magical thinking. However, from around the age of seven, many begin to question these beliefs, reflecting the rise of internal filtering and rationalisation.

NLP and Hypnotherapy Frameworks

Within NLP and Ericksonian hypnotherapy, it is commonly taught that the *Critical Faculty begins forming around the age of 7 and becomes more rigid and protective by 11 or 12.*

This framework is used to explain why childhood is such a critical period for belief formation, and why many limiting beliefs and unconscious patterns originate before the Critical Faculty is strong enough to question them.

Why This Matters in Hypnosis

Understanding the development of the Critical Faculty helps explain:

- why children are more hypnotically suggestible

- why early childhood programming (like negative comments or traumatic experiences) can bypass logical filtering and shape core beliefs

- why hypnosis works so effectively in adults.

The lack of a strong Critical Faculty is why children cannot filter out suggestions and easily accept ideas. If you tell a child there's a monster under the bed, they might believe it completely. If you tell them they are a superhero, they embrace that belief wholeheartedly.

A child will believe you if you say: "You are so brave. You can do anything."

However, if you tell an adult the same thing, they might say, "Hmm, not really. I've never been brave."

That's the Critical Faculty talking.

As we grow older, that filter becomes more rigid. It starts to protect our limitations — even when we're ready to outgrow them.

As adults, we become more skeptical and resistant to change because the Critical Faculty has become rigid. It holds onto existing beliefs even when they don't serve us anymore.

This is why hypnosis is so powerful. It bypasses the Critical Faculty and allows us to install new beliefs and behaviours directly into the unconscious mind.

How Do We Bypass the Critical Faculty?

There are several ways hypnosis helps bypass the Critical Faculty so that new suggestions can take hold:

- **Relaxation and Trance Induction**

The more relaxed you are, the more your critical mind takes a backseat.

Have you ever noticed how, just before you fall asleep, your mind drifts and daydreams? This is a natural hypnotic state where the Critical Faculty is relaxed, allowing suggestions to slip in more easily.

- **Confusion and Overload**

The Critical Faculty gets overwhelmed when faced with too much information.

This is a common technique in Ericksonian hypnosis. We overload the Critical Faculty with indirect language, ambiguity or metaphors until it simply lets go.

> *You can forget to remember or remember to forget … and*
> *somewhere in between, your mind drifts where it needs to go.*

When the Conscious Mind is confused, the Unconscious Mind opens up.

- **Storytelling and Metaphors**

The Critical Faculty resists direct instructions, but loves stories. When we use a metaphor in hypnosis, the Conscious Mind enjoys the story, but the Unconscious Mind receives the message hidden within.

This is why fairy tales, myths and bedtime stories stick with us so deeply — they reach the parts of the mind logic can't touch.

When you hear a metaphor, your Unconscious Mind makes its own connections without the Critical Faculty blocking the message. That's why fables, fairytales and myths have such a lasting impact — they embed deeper meanings without triggering resistance.

- **Emotion and Intensity**

Strong emotions bypass the Critical Faculty completely.

Think of a powerful moment in your life — maybe a first love, a major success or a deep loss. The emotional intensity of that moment locked it into your Unconscious Mind instantly, without conscious thought. Hypnosis can leverage positive emotions to make new suggestions stick.

Sequential vs Simultaneous Processing

Think of the Conscious Mind as having step-by-step thinking. It operates sequentially, one thought at a time.

It's like following a recipe — you measure ingredients, mix them and bake them, all in order.

Now think of the Unconscious Mind as working effortlessly and multitasking. It operates simultaneously, handling multiple tasks at once.

When you're driving a car, you're steering, checking mirrors, pressing pedals and thinking about your day, all at the same time. Hypnosis works by communicating directly with this multi-tasking Unconscious Mind, allowing deep changes to happen without effort.

Final Thought: Why This Matters for You as a Hypnotherapist

When you understand the relationship between the Conscious Mind, Unconscious Mind and Critical Faculty, you're not just learning hypnosis, you're learning how the human mind really works.

This is the key to helping clients:

- quit habits they've struggled with for years

- rewire beliefs that once seemed permanent

- reclaim confidence, joy and peace

- step into powerful new behaviours — effortlessly.

As a hypnotherapist, you are not forcing change. You are inviting the unconscious mind to accept new possibilities.

And once the Critical Faculty steps aside, the door opens and transformation begins.

Chapter 4:

Understanding Trance

The Nature of Trance and Its Everyday Presence

Trance is the foundation of hypnosis and a natural state of mind that we all experience regularly without realising it. Contrary to common misconceptions, a trance is not something strange or mystical; instead, it is a deeply relaxed and focused state that allows for powerful transformation and learning.

To illustrate, think about a time you were lost in thought while doing something familiar. For example, have you ever stepped into an elevator, watched the floor numbers change and suddenly realised you weren't sure which floor you were on? Or perhaps you've driven on a long, open road, listening to music, only to snap back into awareness and realise you've gone miles past your turn. This is trance in action — a state where your Unconscious Mind takes over the task at hand, allowing your Conscious Mind to rest.

One of the most common forms of everyday trance is the television trance. Have you ever been so absorbed in watching a show that you only registered that someone had spoken to you minutes later? In that moment, your Unconscious Mind was fully engaged, taking in images and sounds effortlessly. These examples remind us that trance is a natural, relaxed state we can easily enter and use intentionally for healing, learning and growth.

The Role of Trance in Hypnotherapy

In hypnotherapy, trance is intentionally created to achieve a specific, positive outcome. The difference between everyday trance (like zoning out in front of the TV) and therapeutic trance is purpose and direction. When working with a hypnotherapist, you are guided into trance with the intention of achieving a particular result, whether that is healing, learning a new behaviour or accessing deeper resources within yourself.

A key factor in successful hypnotherapy is rapport. In everyday trance, your rapport may be with a book, a movie or even the road ahead of you. In a therapeutic trance, rapport exists between you and the hypnotherapist. This connection allows your Unconscious Mind to open up, listen and accept beneficial suggestions that lead to meaningful change.

It is also important to recognise that clients often arrive in their own trance. For example, someone caught up in anxiety or self-doubt is already in a trance of their own making. As a hypnotherapist, your first step is to gently guide them out of their existing trance and into a purposeful one based on trust and collaboration.

Experiencing Trance for Yourself

As a practitioner, your effectiveness in guiding others into trance will grow as you gain experience in accessing deeper trance states yourself. In my experience, training hundreds of hypnotherapists, one thing has become consistently clear: the better you are at achieving your own trance states, the more skillful you become at helping others do the same.

People new to hypnosis are often surprised by how normal trance feels. It is a natural state where they remain aware and in control, yet are deeply relaxed and focused. For some, it feels like drifting into a daydream, while for others it resembles the calm just before sleep. What's important is that trance allows the Unconscious Mind to take center stage, where the real work happens.

To deepen your understanding, we will explore suggestibility tests and practical exercises later in the book. These techniques will not only demonstrate the reality of trance but also help you develop your ability to access deeper levels of trance yourself.

Stage Hypnosis vs. Hypnotherapy

Many people associate hypnosis with stage performances, where volunteers act in surprising or silly ways. But there's more to this than meets the eye. Stage hypnosis works because participants willingly step into trance. Often, they are outgoing individuals who enjoy the spotlight and want to play along. The hypnotist selects participants who are open to suggestion, making the process appear magical.

In hypnotherapy, the experience is entirely different. While stage hypnosis relies on entertainment, therapeutic hypnosis is about creating positive change. As Milton Erickson demonstrated, clients remain fully in control during therapeutic trance. Hypnotherapy uses trance to address specific goals, such as reducing stress, relieving pain or changing unwanted behaviours.

Interestingly, some of the hypnotic phenomena seen in stage hypnosis — like full-body catalepsy or amnesia for suggestions — have significant therapeutic value. For example, someone with chronic back pain might use trance to achieve deep muscular relaxation and alignment, facilitating relief and healing. Similarly, post-hypnotic amnesia can allow healing suggestions to bypass the Conscious Mind and take effect at a deeper level.

Unlike stage hypnosis, the depth of trance required in hypnotherapy varies. For some clients, light trance is all that is needed to achieve powerful results. For others, a deeper trance may be required. As practitioners, our role is to determine what best serves the client.

Trance for Accelerated Learning

One of the most exciting applications of trance is its ability to enhance learning. When you're in trance, your Unconscious Mind is highly receptive to new information while your Conscious Mind rests. I encourage all students to use trance as a tool for absorbing and recalling information effortlessly.

As Ernest Rossi explains in *The Psychobiology of Mind Body Healing*, learning is profoundly influenced by the state in which it occurs. This means that entering a focused, relaxed state — like trance — is one of the most effective ways to learn complex skills, such as hypnosis.

Here is a simple exercise to experience trance for learning:

1. Pick a spot on the wall above eye level and gently focus on it.

2. Allow your eyes to soften as you notice your peripheral vision expand, becoming aware of what you can see to the left and right.

3. As you focus on this spot, allow yourself to relax more deeply, noticing how your breathing slows and your body becomes calm.

4. Maintain this awareness while reading or listening, and allow your Unconscious Mind to absorb the information effortlessly.

We call this the Learning State. It allows you to remain relaxed, focused and receptive, synchronising your mind for optimal learning. Teachers and learners alike can benefit from this powerful state to improve retention and recall.

Assisting Clients into Trance

The role of the hypnotherapist is to guide clients into trance with care and precision. Early hypnotists often used direct, authoritarian approaches: "close your eyes. Relax now." While effective for some, many people respond better to the indirect, permissive style developed by Milton Erickson, an American psychiatrist widely regarded as the most influential hypnotherapist of the twentieth century. Erickson's conversational techniques, metaphors and ambiguous language patterns encourage the Unconscious Mind to engage naturally.

In this book, you'll be introduced to both direct and indirect approaches, enabling you to adapt to each client's needs. Whether the goal is relaxation, healing or transformation, trance is the gateway to working with the Unconscious Mind.

A Final Thought on Trance

Trance is a natural and powerful tool for learning, growth and change. By mastering your own ability to enter and guide others into trance, you unlock the full potential of the mind. Whether you are learning, healing or helping others, trance is the key to transformation.

Enjoy the process. As you continue reading and practising, you'll find that the more you learn about trance, the more you will experience its benefits for yourself and those you work with.

Chapter 5:

Understanding Brainwaves in Hypnosis

How Your Brain's Frequencies Shape Trance, Transformation and Healing

As a hypnotherapist, one of the most powerful things you should understand is how the brain works, and, more specifically, how the brain's electrical activity changes during hypnosis.

It's easy to think of hypnosis as 'just' relaxation, but there's actually a lot more happening behind the scenes. Your client's brain is shifting gears — moving from one brainwave frequency to another. And as you learn how to work with these frequencies, your ability to create real and lasting change grows exponentially.

Let's dive into the fascinating world of brainwaves and how they relate to trance and healing.

What Are Brainwaves?

Your brain is constantly active. Even when you're asleep, it's sending electrical signals from one neuron to another. These signals create brainwaves, which can be measured by how fast they're firing — called their frequency.

Brainwave frequencies are measured in Hertz (Hz), which simply means cycles per second.

Different brainwave states are associated with different levels of consciousness. In hypnosis, we're particularly interested in slowing the brain down — helping a client move from the fast-paced, analytical thinking of waking life into deeper, slower, more receptive states.

Let's take a look at the five main brainwave frequencies you'll hear about in hypnosis.

Brainwave ranges are not rigid compartments but overlapping patterns that reflect how the brain is functioning in a given moment.

Gamma Waves (above 40 Hz)

- **State:** super-conscious, peak mental processing

- **When It Happens**: high-level problem solving, complex learning, spiritual insight

- **Relevance to Hypnosis:** rare in trance — this is the brain on high alert and may be seen during moments of insight or breakthrough.

Beta Waves (13 – 30 Hz)

- **State:** alert, awake, logical thinking

- **When It Happens**: working, talking, analysing, worrying, planning

- **Relevance to Hypnosis:** Beta is where your client starts — it's their usual 'conscious state'. But Beta is also where resistance lives. The Critical Faculty is most active here. To access the unconscious mind, we must guide the client down into a slower, more receptive frequency.

Alpha Waves (8 – 12 Hz)

- **State:** relaxed, focused, inward attention

- **When It Happens:** daydreaming, light meditation, the moment just before sleep

- **Relevance to Hypnosis:** Alpha is the gateway to trance. This is where the Critical Faculty begins to relax. The client becomes more open to suggestion, more imaginative and more receptive.

Think of Alpha as standing at the door of the Unconscious Mind. Once here, you can knock gently and be invited in.

Theta Waves (4 – 7 Hz)

- **State:** deep trance, unconscious access, emotional memory

- **When It Happens:** deep meditation, hypnosis, REM sleep

- **Relevance to Hypnosis:** Theta is where much of the change work happens. This is the zone where long-held beliefs, emotional patterns and unconscious programs can be accessed and updated.

This is why your suggestions are so powerful during hypnosis — the Conscious Mind has stepped aside, and the Unconscious is listening.

Delta Waves (0.5 – 4 Hz)

- **State:** deep, dreamless sleep

- **When It Happens**: slow-wave sleep, deep unconscious states

- **Relevance to Hypnosis:** not common in standard hypnotherapy, but in healing trance or during regression work, clients may dip into Delta briefly. The body is healing. The unconscious is deeply at work.

The Trance Journey: From Beta to Theta

When you guide a client into hypnosis, you're helping their brain shift states:

- They arrive in Beta — alert, perhaps a little nervous.

- As you speak in a calm, rhythmic voice, they begin to relax into Alpha.

- Through deepening techniques, they drift down into Theta — where deep change happens.

- You guide the work and then gently bring them back up through Alpha to Beta, refreshed and changed.

Why Hypnotherapists Must Understand Brainwaves

Understanding brainwaves gives you a kind of X-ray vision for the hypnotic process. You'll start to notice what state your client is in — not just from their body language or breathing, but by sensing what frequency their brain might be operating in.

Here's why this matters:

- When a client is in Beta, they might resist your suggestions.

- When they drop into Alpha, the door to the unconscious begins to open.

- In Theta, the unconscious accepts new ideas, healing and beliefs.

- And if a client slips into Delta, you may need to lighten the trance slightly to bring them back into a responsive state.

The Brain's Natural Patterns and Hypnosis

It's also worth knowing that your brain cycles through these states naturally, several times per day.

- You drift into Alpha when daydreaming or walking in nature.

- You enter Theta as you fall asleep or just before waking up.

- You cycle through Delta during the night.

So when you hypnotise someone, you're not doing something 'unnatural' — you're simply guiding them into a state their brain already knows - on purpose, for a purpose.

Final Thought: Brainwaves are the Bridge

Brainwaves are the bridge between the Conscious and Unconscious Minds. As a hypnotherapist, the more you understand this, the more you can:

- know where your client is in the trance process

- tailor your language and deepeners effectively

- recognise signs of resistance or receptivity

- deliver change suggestions at the optimal moment

- feel confident that you're working with the brain's natural rhythms — not against them

Bonus Exercise: Tuning In to Brainwaves

The next time you guide someone into trance, imagine their brainwaves gently slowing:

- from busy, chattering Beta

- to calm, flowing Alpha

- into deep, receptive Theta

Feel that shift as if you were tuning a radio dial — click by click, the frequency changes. You're not forcing. You're guiding. You're allowing the mind to soften, the body to relax and the door to open.

That's the art of hypnosis. And now you understand the science too.

Chapter 6:

Hypnotic Rapport — The Invisible Bridge to the Unconscious Mind

I f there's one skill that will change every client session, every conversation, every moment of connection you have, it's rapport.

Have you ever sat with someone and just felt like you were on the same wavelength? You didn't need to think about what to say; you just clicked. You were comfortable, in tune and, somehow, they just got you.

That's rapport. And in hypnosis, it's everything.

Would you like to give hypnotic suggestions that are accepted effortlessly by the client's Unconscious Mind?

Would it help if clients felt instantly comfortable and safe with you — even before formal hypnosis begins?

Would you like to naturally guide someone into trance just by how you speak, move and breathe?

That's what hypnotic rapport makes possible.

The Power of Connection Beyond Words

Hypnosis is not something we do to someone, it's something we do with someone. For that to happen, there must be trust — not just logical trust, but unconscious alignment. Rapport is how we get there.

In fact, you could say rapport is the bridge that links the Conscious and Unconscious Minds — both yours and your client's. It allows you to speak in a way that bypasses resistance and lets the Unconscious Mind say, "Yes. I trust you. I'll go there with you."

Without rapport, a suggestion might bounce off the Conscious Mind like a pebble on armour. With rapport, a suggestion can melt resistance, slipping beneath awareness and planting the seeds of change.

Rapport is a state of trust, connection, and unconscious alignment between you and another person. In NLP, we define it as:

> *Responsiveness in communication via matching and mirroring someone so they accept, uncritically, the suggestions you give them*

In other words:

- they follow your lead

- they respond without resistance

- their unconscious mind says yes.

This isn't manipulation. This is deep alignment.

In hypnosis, this is how we begin. Rapport is the induction before the induction.

The Science and Structure Behind Rapport

Here's where it gets fascinating. You've likely heard that 93% of communication is non-verbal. Let's unpack that.

This idea comes from a body of research often attributed to psychologist Albert Mehrabian. In the 1970s, Mehrabian identified that when it comes to emotional meaning:

- 55% is conveyed through physiology — our posture, gestures and facial expressions

- 38% comes from tonality — how we say what we say

- only 7% comes from the actual words.

Mehrabian's findings specifically pertain to situations where there is a mismatch between verbal and non-verbal cues, such as when someone says they're fine, but their tone and posture suggest otherwise. In such cases, people tend to trust the non-verbal signals over the words spoken. His research applies specifically to the communication of feelings and attitudes, but in hypnosis — where we work directly with feelings and unconscious states — this model is deeply relevant.

If words are only 7% of emotional meaning, why do we place so much focus on language in hypnosis?

The answer is that this 7% is everything when the Unconscious Mind is listening. In turn, that brings us to something vital …

Why NLP is Essential in Hypnosis

We say it proudly: linguistics is our middle name.

In Neuro-Linguistic Programming, language is not just vocabulary; it's how we code reality. And, in hypnosis, language becomes a doorway into change.

Physiology and tone create rapport. If you're a hypnotherapist and you're not paying attention to what's happening beyond the words, you're missing over 90% of the message. But it's the words — those well-chosen suggestions, metaphors, presuppositions and hypnotic patterns — that guide the unconscious mind to change.

Think of it like this: Your physiology gets you through the front door. Your tone keeps you in the room. Your words are what rearranges the furniture.

As a hypnotherapist, you must learn how to use language artfully, intentionally and with precision. NLP gives you the tools to do just that.

Understanding the 7% — the words — is just as critical as understanding the other 93% because the words you use aren't just heard — they're felt. And, when combined with physiology and tonality in a state of rapport, these words become transformational.

So while words are 'only 7%' of communication, in hypnosis and NLP we make them count – subtly, elegantly and unconsciously.

Rapport in Practice — Match, Mirror, Connect

Let's turn theory into practice.

In NLP, we do something special: we denominalise rapport. We turn it from a vague idea into a precise, repeatable process. Rapport isn't about liking someone. It's about being like them because people like people who are like themselves.

Match and Mirror

Rapport is built by matching and mirroring in terms of physiology, tonality and language.

Physiology makes up 55% of communication. It includes posture, gestures, head tilt, facial expressions, blinking and breathing.

- Posture: are they upright or relaxed; leaning in or sitting back?

- Gesture: are they expressive or still?

- Facial expressions and blinking rate: are they smiling, squinting or tense?

- Breathing: Fast, slow, chest-based, belly-based?

Tonality makes up 38% of communication. It includes pitch, tempo, timbre (voice quality) and volume.

- Pitch: high or low?

- Tempo: fast or slow?

- Timbre: warm, crisp, soft, smooth?

- Volume: loud, soft, confident or hesitant?

Language makes up 7% of communication. It includes key words, representational systems (visual/auditory/kinesthetic), rhythms and chunk size.

When someone crosses their arms, you do the same — gently. If they lean forward, you do too. If they breathe slowly, you begin to match that rhythm.

In doing so, you're sending the unconscious message: 'I'm like you. I understand you. You can trust me.'

And here's the key: when rapport is strong, you can lead. That's what makes it so powerful in hypnosis. When you change your posture or breathing, your client will begin to follow — unconsciously.

That's pacing and leading. The ratio is usually 3:1 and it's how we guide someone into trance, change and transformation.

Crossover Mirroring

What if someone is in a highly anxious or agitated state and you don't want to join them in that energy? You can still build rapport using crossover mirroring. For example, if their leg is shaking, you might tap your finger at the same speed, gradually slowing the tapping until they begin to settle.

It's subtle. It's elegant. It's masterful.

Intonation Patterns — How Your Voice Shapes Unconscious Response

Beyond pitch, speed and volume lies something even more nuanced, intonation. This is the rise and fall of your voice as you speak, and it matters — especially in hypnosis.

Different intonation patterns create different unconscious effects. For example:

- Falling tone (Command Tone) ↘ suggests completion, certainty and authority. "You can go deeper now ↘"

- Rising tone (Question Tone) ↗ implies curiosity, openness or a question. "And I wonder what you'll notice next ↗"

- Level tone (Statement Tone) → often draws the listener into a trance-like rhythm. "That's right ... just like that ... continuing to relax →"

Your intonation patterns influence how your words land. The main tones used in hypnosis are the Statement (Level) Tone and the Command (Falling) Tone. If used incorrectly, the Question (Rising) Tone can make you sound unsure or as if you are seeking permission.

For example, if you say, "You'll feel calm and confident now" with a questioning tone, the suggestion dissolves. But if you say, "You'll feel calm and confident now" with a firm, grounded command tone, the unconscious mind will take it in.

In therapy, learning to listen to a client's natural intonation — and gently match it — builds powerful rapport. Knowing how to lead with intentional intonation allows you to soften resistance and deliver suggestions more effectively.

Imagine you're speaking with a potential client over the phone, and they ask, "How much do you charge?"

If you respond with a questioning (rising) tone ("I charge $200 per session?") this may convey uncertainty, leading the client to doubt your confidence.

However, if you respond with a confident tone ("I charge $200 per session") the assertive delivery will communicate confidence and professionalism, making the client more likely to trust and engage with you.

Remember: clients don't just buy your services — they buy your certainty.

Try this: practice saying the same sentence with different intonations and notice how your body — and the listener's body — responds. That's the magic of hypnotic communication; it's not just what you say, but how you say it.

What Becomes Possible When You Master Rapport

Rapport isn't something you do to someone, it's something you create with someone.

When done right:

- clients relax before trance even begins

- suggestions land without resistance

- transformation flows naturally.

Best of all, you'll feel it.

You'll feel when you and your client are in sync. Rapport is more than a skill. It's a state. It's the foundation of all powerful communication, especially in hypnosis. You cannot take someone deep into transformation without first meeting them at the unconscious level.

Next time you greet a client, notice:

- their posture

- their tone

- their words

- their energy.

And, with subtle grace, join them there. Once you join them, you can lead them to where they want to go.

If you've ever wondered what makes a hypnotherapist stand out, it's not fancy scripts. It's not clever techniques. It's their ability to connect — deeply, authentically and unconsciously.

That's the power of hypnotic rapport.

Chapter 7:

Sensory Acuity — Seeing What Others Miss

Imagine being able to look at someone — really look — and know exactly how they're feeling, even when they haven't said a word. Imagine noticing the moment your client shifts state — even before they realise it themselves. That's the gift of sensory acuity.

In NLP and hypnosis, this skill isn't just useful, it's essential.

Why Sensory Acuity Matters in Change Work

Let's start with a couple of questions:

When you're communicating with a client, wouldn't you like to know whether your message is landing the way you intend?

Wouldn't it be useful to see, with absolute clarity, when your client agrees, when they hesitate, when they withdraw and when they lean in — not with words but with their unconscious signals?

Sensory acuity gives you that. It gives you access to your client's real-time inner world through external micro-signals in their physiology.

In other words, it helps you tell what's happening on the inside by watching what's happening on the outside.

If you're a coach, therapist or trainer — or even a parent or leader — this ability allows you to flex your communication, adapt your approach and connect more deeply.

It helps you respond, rather than assume.

What is Sensory Acuity?

Sensory acuity is the art and science of observing minute changes in a person's physiology and recognising that those changes have meaning.

It's not about mind-reading. It's about sensory awareness.

If your client's skin tone shifts, their breathing pattern changes or the size of their lower lip alters slightly, these aren't random movements. They're reflections of internal state changes.

When your sensory acuity is trained, you no longer miss these signals. You know when to continue, when to shift gears and when to say nothing at all.

The Legacy of Milton Erickson

Sensory acuity was modelled into NLP from the brilliant hypnotist Milton H. Erickson, who was legendary for his ability to notice the tiniest physical cues. In fact, Erickson's acuity was so finely tuned that he could detect a patient's pulse by watching their ankle.

How did he develop that level of observation?

Through necessity.

Erickson contracted polio at age 17, which left him nearly paralyzed. While bedridden, he closely observed the movement of infants and others learning to walk, studied subtle shifts in muscle and balance, and used mental imagery of those movements (his 'body memory') to gradually re-educate his own musculature.

He observed every movement, every muscle shift and every change in balance. Then he taught himself to walk again using that model.

That level of observation became one of the foundational skills in hypnosis and NLP.

The Five Elements of Sensory Acuity

To build sensory acuity, we begin by learning to calibrate. We observe what someone's baseline state looks like and then notice when it changes.

There are five key elements we need to pay attention to:

- Skin colour — look for subtle changes, especially in the face, neck and upper chest. Colour may shift from light to dark or vice versa, regardless of skin tone.

- Skin tonus (muscle tension) — the tightness or looseness of facial muscles can signal changes in emotion or internal processing. You'll notice this most clearly through the way light reflects on the skin: taut muscles create shine; relaxed muscles absorb it.

- Breathing — watch both the location (chest, diaphragm, belly) and rate (fast and shallow vs slow and deep). One of the best ways to detect shifts in breathing is to match it subtly. When breath changes, you'll feel it.

- Lower lip size — it really does change! When blood flows into the lower lip, it appears fuller and smoother. When blood drains out, it becomes thinner and more lined. These changes reflect shifts in emotional or physiological state.

- Eyes and pupil size — are the eyes focused or unfocused? Are pupils dilated or constricted? When someone 'goes inside' to access a memory or emotion, the eyes will often lose focus or shift direction.

Tip: Use your peripheral vision. Rather than staring intently, soften your focus and observe the entire field of the person. This allows you to take in breathing, movement, posture and micro-changes all at once, without being invasive.

Observation Without Judgement

This is important: sensory acuity is not body language and it is not mind-reading.

Those old body language charts from the 90s — 'crossed arms = defensive' — are too generic and often inaccurate. That posture might mean someone is cold or comfortable, or simply that they habitually cross their arms.

Context matters. In sensory acuity, you don't guess; you observe and you build a baseline through calibration.

Calibration — The Key to Sensory Acuity

Calibration simply means learning to notice and measure the changes in another person's physiology in a reliable way. Think of it as tuning in to someone's 'baseline signals' so that when those signals shift, you can recognise the change.

- Baseline: you first ask questions to elicit known states and watch what the body does when that state is accessed (For example, 'Think of someone or something that you like/dislike', 'Tell me about a time you felt happy', 'What's 2+2?'). While they answer, you observe their breathing, skin tone, posture, micro-expressions and voice.

- Compare: once you know what their physiology looks like in those states, when you see that same physiology again, you'll know what state is likely present.

- No guessing: this way, you're not assuming or mind-reading, you're measuring change against a baseline you've already established.

Calibration is like tuning a radio. At first, it's static. You adjust the dial until the station comes in clearly. Once you've tuned to the right frequency, you'll always recognise it again. With people, once you've tuned in to their 'frustrated signal' or 'relaxed signal,' you can spot it whenever it shows up.

Why Calibration Matters

Calibration keeps you objective, rather than making assumptions. It shows you in real time whether your communication is landing. It lets you adapt instantly — to challenge, soften or deepen your approach.

Calibration in Action

If a client talks about something frustrating and their breathing moves up to the chest and their skin tone reddens, that's a snapshot of their frustration physiology. Later, if they show that same physiology, you know something in your communication has activated a similar state and you can adjust accordingly.

That's what makes calibration the cornerstone of flexible communication.

Learning the Art of Acuity

Acuity isn't something you master by theory. You develop it by doing.

Here's an example of a simple partner exercise you can do with a friend, family member or colleague:

- Sit at a 45° angle to your partner so you can observe breathing.

- Ask them to think about something they deeply enjoy. Observe. Calibrate.

- Clear the state.

- Ask them to think about something they dislike. Observe. Calibrate.

- Repeat.

- Finally, ask them to think of either something they enjoy or dislike. Your job is to guess which state they're accessing based on their physiology alone.

You'll be amazed at what you notice when you truly pay attention.

What Becomes Possible When You Master This Skill

When you sharpen your sensory acuity, you become a more powerful communicator. You're more precise, more attuned and more intuitive.

You'll notice micro-signals that others miss. You'll respond more effectively. You'll know when to challenge, when to soften and when to pause.

It all starts by learning to see.

Chapter 8:

The Three 'F's: Feel, Felt, Found – A Powerful Tool for Trust and Rapport in Hypnosis

In hypnosis, building trust and rapport with a client is one of the most essential skills. Without trust, a client may resist going into trance or may question the suggestions given. This is where the Three 'F's – Feel, Felt, Found come into play.

The Feel-Felt-Found framework is a simple yet powerful conversational technique used to validate a client's experience, build rapport and gently guide them toward a new perspective. It is particularly effective in pre-talk, during suggestion work and in reframing resistance in hypnosis.

Why Use the Three 'F's?

There are four key reasons you would use the Feel-Felt-Found framework:

- Validation: the framework acknowledges the client's current emotional state, showing empathy and understanding

- Connection: the framework helps clients feel heard and accepted, which increases trust.

- Transformation: using the framework allows the client to see that others have had similar experiences and have successfully moved forward.

- Indirect suggestion: instead of directly challenging a client's belief, the framework subtly introduces a possibility for change.

This technique is a valuable pre-hypnosis tool that makes induction and suggestion work smoother.

How to Use the Three 'F's in Hypnosis

The formula is simple:

- **Feel** – acknowledge and validate their experience.

- **Felt** – relate their experience to others or yourself, showing they are not alone.

- **Found** – offer a solution or positive outcome they can consider.

This can be used at various points in a hypnosis session:

- Before induction (to address doubts or fears about hypnosis)

- During trance work (to embed suggestions)

- In post-hypnotic reinforcement (to ensure lasting change)

Breaking Down the Three 'F's in Hypnosis

Here are the three components of the framework in more detail.

FEEL – Validating the Client's Experience

People want to feel heard and understood. Before guiding someone into a trance, it's essential to validate their current feelings — without assuming or claiming that you fully understand their experience.

In hypnosis and NLP, we avoid using phrases like 'I understand how you feel' because no one can truly understand another person's unique experience. Instead, we pace the client's reality by acknowledging what they feel is perfectly natural, normal and acceptable.

This respectful validation helps to quickly establish rapport and trust, making it much easier for the unconscious mind to feel safe enough to relax and engage fully in the hypnotic process.

By acknowledging what they FEEL, you lower their resistance and make them feel safe.

FELT – Normalising Their Experience

Once the client feels heard and validated, the next step is to normalise what they're experiencing. This is done by letting them know that others have FELT the same way — and that what they are feeling is not unusual nor a sign that something is wrong.

When you let a client know that many others have FELT similar emotions — whether it's uncertainty, nervousness, skepticism or even curiosity — it immediately reduces feelings of isolation. They realise, often with a sense of relief, that their reactions are completely normal and that they are not the 'only one' feeling this way.

This simple statement can have a huge impact because it connects their experience to a wider human experience — and reassures their unconscious mind that it's safe to continue.

In short, validation opens the door and normalisation invites them to step through it with confidence.

This stage creates connection — they begin to relate to others who have had similar feelings but successfully moved forward.

FOUND – Providing a Path to Resolution

Now that the client feels heard (Feel) and knows that others have shared similar experiences (Felt), the final step is to introduce a positive outcome — by showing them what others have discovered after moving forward.

This is where you plant a seed of hope and possibility.

You are not telling the client what will happen to them personally — you are simply sharing what others have FOUND after relaxing, trusting the process and allowing themselves to experience hypnosis fully.

This step is incredibly important because it subtly opens a future direction for the client's Unconscious Mind, creating an expectation that positive change is not only possible but that it's already happening for people just like them.

It's important to remember that you're not making promises or guarantees. You're offering evidence — the collective experiences of others —so the client can imagine themselves finding success too, without pressure.

In short, FOUND is about creating a bridge from where they are now to where they could very naturally go simply by following the process.

This stage opens their mind to possibility and change. It subtly shifts their focus toward a new belief without forcing it.

Putting It All Together

Here are some examples of pre-talk.

Example for Client Skepticism

Clients may wonder if they can actually be hypnotised or whether hypnosis will work for them. In these cases, try: "it makes perfect sense that you might *feel* that way. Many people I've worked with have *felt* the same way at first. What they *found* is that once they relaxed and allowed themselves to simply follow the process, they were able to experience incredible changes — often more easily than they expected."

Example for Anxiety or Fear

Try this if your client is nervous or hesitant: "It's completely natural to *feel* uncertain about this process. I've had many clients who have *felt* uncertain about trying something new. And what they *found* is that hypnosis helped them feel calmer, more in control and capable of handling situations with ease."

Example for Fear of Losing Control

Clients may be worried about the loss of control. If so, try this: "It's very natural to *feel* concerned about loss of control. Many people I've worked with have *felt* the same way. And what they *found* is that hypnosis actually gave them more control — over their thoughts, emotions and behaviours — in ways they hadn't experienced before."

Example for "I Tried Hypnosis Before and It Didn't Work"

Try this if your client has had a previous experience with hypnosis that wasn't positive: "It makes perfect sense to *feel* cautious if you've had a previous experience that didn't meet your expectations. Many clients have *felt* that way after trying hypnosis elsewhere. And what they *found*, when we worked together, is that with the right approach, they were able to experience real, meaningful changes."

Example for "I'm Not Sure I Can Be Hypnotised"

Try this if your client is a little ambivalent about whether they can be hypnotised: "It's very normal to *feel* unsure about whether hypnosis will work for you. Many people I've worked with have *felt* the same way. And what they *found* is that hypnosis is about simply following the process, and they drifted into trance much more easily than they ever expected."

Example for Feeling Nervous About "Letting Go"

Some clients may feel awkward about 'letting go'. If so, try this: "It's completely natural to *feel* a little nervous about letting go and trusting the process. A lot of people I've worked with have *felt* that same hesitancy at first. What they *found* is that in hypnosis, you actually stay fully in charge while allowing your Unconscious Mind to gently guide you towards the changes you truly want."

Each of these examples:

- starts by pacing their emotional reality (Feel)

- Normalises their experience (Felt)

- Leads to a positive outcome, without force (Found)

Using Feel-Felt-Found During Hypnosis

This technique isn't just for pre-talk; it can be woven into the hypnosis session itself.

Example: Overcoming a Limiting Belief

Imagine a client who struggles with self-confidence: "I know that right now, you may *feel* like confidence is something other people have, but not you. Many people have *felt* the same way, believing they would never be truly confident. But what they have *found* is that as they began to tap into their inner strengths, they naturally created a deep and lasting sense of confidence."

Here, we are embedding a reframe into their Unconscious Mind.

Using Feel-Felt-Found for Resistance During Hypnosis

Some clients may resist suggestions if they seem too different from their current beliefs. Instead of arguing, use Feel-Felt-Found to gently nudge them toward change.

Example: Client Resisting Weight Loss Suggestions

Let's say you're working with a client who struggles to believe they can change their habits and maintain a healthy lifestyle: "It's completely natural to *feel* that staying motivated with healthy eating has been a struggle. Many people have *felt* the same way. But what they *found* is that once they began tuning into their body's natural signals, making healthier choices became easy ... and even enjoyable."

By doing this, you are redirecting their thoughts without directly contradicting their beliefs.

Practising the Three 'F's

To integrate this into your hypnosis work, practice formulating Feel-Felt-Found responses in different situations.

- Write down common objections or fears clients might have.

- Use the Three F's to craft a response.

- Practise saying it naturally and smoothly.

- Apply it in real sessions and observe how it builds rapport.

Final Thoughts

The Three 'F's – Feel, Felt, Found is one of the simple yet powerful tools for overcoming resistance, deepening rapport and gently guiding clients toward transformation.

By using this approach consistently, you will:

- gain instant trust and rapport with clients

- reduce resistance to hypnosis and suggestions

- make clients feel understood and supported

- help clients embrace new possibilities without feeling forced.

Start using Feel-Felt-Found today and watch how it transforms your effectiveness as a hypnotist.

Chapter 9:

Personal History and Effective Questioning

The Importance of Personal History in Hypnotherapy

Every successful hypnotherapy session begins with understanding your client's personal history. Gathering information about your client's presenting problem and the events that led up to it is not just about collecting data — it is about establishing trust, clarity and rapport. A well-executed personal history sets the foundation for effective intervention, ensuring your sessions achieve the desired results.

Equally important is knowing how to ask the right questions and interpret the answers using tools like the Meta Model from NLP. These techniques will help you clarify vague or distorted information, uncover the root cause of the client's issue and identify where the client may feel stuck in their life.

In addition, you will learn Krasner's structured process to follow to ensure that even beginners can conduct a successful hypnotherapy session.

Effective Questioning Techniques

At the start of a session, your role is to ask clear, focused questions to:

- identify the presenting problem

- uncover patterns or root causes

- build rapport and demonstrate understanding.

The questions below will help you build a complete picture of your client's situation. Pay attention not only to their answers but also to how they answer. Are they at cause (feeling in control of their life), or are they at effect (feeling controlled by external forces)?

Questions for Gathering Personal History

1. Why are you here? Why else? Why else?

- *Elicit all the reasons the client has come to you.*

2. How do you know you have this problem?

- *Identify their internal strategy and any external diagnoses/labels.*

3. How long have you had the problem? Was there a time when you didn't have it? What have you done about it?

- *Explore the timeline and previous attempts to resolve it.*

4. What happened the first time you had the problem? What emotions were present?

- *Pinpoint the root cause and associated emotional triggers.*

5. What events have happened since then? What emotions were present?

- *Trace the problem's development and its emotional impact/charge.*

6. What is the relationship between these events and your current situation in life?

- *Identify recurring patterns and past experiences, and links to the present-day issue.*

7. Tell me about your parents, siblings or key relationships. How do these relationships connect to your current situation?

- *Explore family dynamics, relational influence and patterns.*

8. Tell me about your childhood in relationship to this problem.

- *Uncover any early experiences that may have shaped their beliefs.*

9. Is there a purpose for having this problem? Ask your Unconscious Mind.

- *Encourage reflection and deeper exploration – introspection and unconscious insight.*

10. When did you choose to have this situation created? Why? Ask your Unconscious Mind.

- *Empower the client to take responsibility/ownership for resolving it.*

11. Is there something your Unconscious Mind wants you to know that would allow the problem to disappear?

- *Connect directly to the Unconscious for insight and inner guidance.*

12. Is it okay with your Unconscious Mind to support us in removing this problem today?

- *Establishes readiness for change and gain permission to proceed with the session.*

13. How will you know when this problem has totally disappeared?

- *What will you be seeing, hearing, feeling or saying to yourself when the problem has disappeared?*

Using the Meta Model: Precision Questioning

As clients describe their issues, they delete, distort or generalise information — often unconsciously. The Meta Model is an NLP tool designed to help you:

- recover specific details hidden by vague statements

- challenge distortions or limiting beliefs

- clarify generalisations to uncover deeper truths.

For example:

- If a client says, "Nobody listens to me," you might ask: "Nobody? Can you think of one person who does listen to you?"

- If a client says, "He makes me angry," you could ask: "How does what he does lead to you choosing to feel angry?"

By asking Meta Model questions, you encourage the client to think critically and access information they may not have consciously considered.

The Meta Model is studied in depth during NLP Practitioner and NLP Master Practitioner Trainings. You will learn how to use these patterns fluently to uncover specific details, challenge unhelpful beliefs and guide clients to clarity and empowerment.

Krasner's Steps to a Successful Hypnotherapy Session

Integrating Dr A.M. Krasner's method of hypnotherapy provides a structure to guide you through a complete and effective hypnotherapy session. Here is how we teach Krasner's method in a clear and simple 8-step process, adapted for our philosophy and style.

1. Demystify Hypnosis (expanded in Chapter 10 – Pre-Talk & Suggestibility Tests)

Many clients arrive with misconceptions or fears about hypnosis. It's essential to demystify the process to create trust and safety.

Explain that:

- Trance is natural. "Hypnosis is simply a natural state of focused attention, like when you're completely absorbed in a movie or daydreaming, reading or watching TV."

- All hypnosis is self-hypnosis - you're simply guiding the client to use their own mind more effectively.

- Intelligent people make great subjects. Hypnosis requires focus, not gullibility.

- Don't expect to feel hypnotised but do expect to feel very relaxed.

- A person can emerge at any time. They are always in control.

At this stage, also address any concerns or questions the client has to set their mind at ease. The three F's from Chapter 8 are useful here to validate, normalise and solve any fears and misconceptions about hypnosis.

When clients understand these truths, they relax and trust in the process begins.

2. Explain Hypnosis

Explain what hypnosis is, how it works and why it is so effective. Use simple metaphors and visualisations to make it easy for beginners to understand.

For example:

- "Think of your mind like an iceberg. Your Conscious Mind is the tip above water, but your Unconscious Mind is the massive part below—it runs your habits, emotions, and automatic behaviors. Hypnosis allows us to communicate directly with the Unconscious to create change."

- Bypass of the Critical Faculty (see Chapter 3 - bypassing the critical faculty section)

- It's the accepting of selective thinking, thoughts, concepts and ideas that are OK by you and consistent with your values - you will not do anything that is against your values or morals.

- Let the client know it's simply using the power of their intelligence, focus and imagination, and following your instructions.

Visual metaphors are a wonderful way to help clients understand the process of hypnosis and how lasting changes occur at the Unconscious level. Beginners can use these metaphors as simple stories or explanations to illustrate how hypnosis works. One effective metaphor is the garden metaphor.

The Garden Metaphor

Imagine the Unconscious Mind as a fertile garden where seeds can grow into strong, thriving plants. The seeds represent thoughts, beliefs and habits. In this session, we are planting new, positive seeds of suggestion that will grow into healthy behaviours, thoughts and feelings.

We remove any weeds — the limiting beliefs or unwanted behaviours — that no longer serve you. And, just as a gardener tends to their plants with care, your Unconscious Mind will nurture these new suggestions so they flourish and become part of your life.

By using visual metaphors like the garden, beginners can easily explain the process in a way that feels natural and reassuring to clients. These metaphors also provide the client with an engaging mental image that deepens their connection to the hypnosis process.

Step 2 is to reinforce that hypnosis is safe, comfortable and collaborative. You and your client are partners in the process, working together toward their desired outcome.

3. The Interview

The interview is where you gather information about the client's presenting problem, what they want to change and what their goals are.

Use the questions for gathering personal history outlined earlier in this chapter to uncover:

- the root of the problem

- the client's beliefs and emotional triggers

- what success or resolution looks like to them.

As you ask the questions, listen carefully and write their answers verbatim. These words are gold and your roadmap to meaningful therapy.

4. Suggestibility Tests (expanded in the following chapter)

Suggestibility tests are designed to demonstrate the hypnotic process to the client while also allowing you to gauge their responsiveness. These simple demonstrations build confidence and show how easily the mind can respond to suggestion.

Here are a few beginner-friendly suggestibility tests:

a) The Bucket and Balloon Test

Ask the client to hold both arms out straight with their hands closed like a fist. Say, *"In a moment, I want you to imagine a heavy bucket full of sand being placed in your left hand, pulling it down ... while your right hand feels lighter and lighter as though a helium balloon is gently lifting it up into the air."* Observe the response — their hands may move naturally, providing a tangible example of suggestibility.

b) The Magnetic Fingers Test

Ask the client to clasp their hands together, extend their index fingers and hold them about an inch apart. Say, *"Imagine there's an invisible magnet pulling your fingers closer and closer together ... the more you resist, the stronger the magnetic pull becomes."* Most clients will notice their fingers moving closer together, which builds their belief in the process.

c) The Finger Vice Test

Ask the client to clasp their hands together, bend their elbows, extend their index fingers and hold them about an inch apart in front of their eyes. Then ask them to imagine their fingers are coming together and being locked together as if squeezed by a vice. Say, *"The more you try to pull them apart, the more tightly they stick together ... as if they're glued in place."*

d) The Body Rotation Test:

Ask the client to stand with their feet hip-width apart, facing forward. Give the following instructions: *"Raise your right hand, point your index finger and slowly turn to the right as far as you can without moving your feet. Take a mental note of how far you've gone, and then return to the front. Now, close your eyes and imagine yourself turning again ... but this time, picture yourself going much farther—almost 360 degrees—as though your body can stretch and twist more easily than ever before."*

After the visualisation, have the client physically repeat the action. They will almost always turn farther than before, demonstrating how we can overcome physical limits by engaging the Unconscious Mind. Say, *"Notice how much farther you went this time ... it's amazing how powerful your mind can be when you allow yourself to imagine new possibilities."*

These simple yet powerful tests build the client's confidence in the hypnotic process and give you feedback on how to adjust your approach during the session.

5. Hypnotic Induction

The induction is where you formally guide the client into a relaxed state of trance. This can be done through visualisation, storytelling or direct instructions.

For example, you might say, *"Focus on a spot on the wall above eye level. As you breathe in and out, allow your body to relax more deeply with each breath ... your eyes might feel heavy ... and when you're ready, you can close them and let go."*

Inductions can be gentle and permissive or more structured, depending on the client.

6. Convincers

Convincers provide the client with clear, tangible evidence that they are in a state of trance. This builds their belief in the process and deepens their receptivity.

For example, you might say, *"Notice that your hand feels as though it is stuck to your chair ... the more you try to move it, the more it stays in place."*

Convincers could also include arm catalepsy (where the arm remains stiff) or suggestions of heaviness or lightness in the body.

7. Therapy/Hypnotic Suggestions (see Chapter 17 to write effective suggestions using SPARK)

Once the client is in trance, deliver tailored suggestions that address their presenting problem. These suggestions should reflect the goals and outcomes discussed during the interview.

An example for stress relief may be: *"From now on, every time you take a deep breath, a wave of calm and relaxation will flow through your body, allowing you to feel more at ease."*

Whereas an example for smoking cessation may sound like: *"Each time you see a cigarette, you will feel a deep sense of satisfaction knowing you are free and a permanent fresh-air breather."*

Suggestions can be embedded within stories, metaphors or direct statements, depending on what works best for the client.

8. Emerging

Gently bring the client back to full awareness and conclude the session.

For example, you might say: *"In a moment, I will count from one to five. As I count, you will feel more awake, refreshed, and energised. One ... feeling calm. Two ... starting to notice the room. Three ... bringing back a sense of clarity. Four ... becoming more aware. And five ... open your eyes, feeling wonderful."*

After emerging, take a few moments to review the session with the client, reinforcing the positive changes and answering any questions they may have.

Bringing It All Together

When you combine precise questioning techniques, the Meta Model and Krasner's 8 steps , you will have a clear and effective framework for every hypnotherapy session.

For beginners, this structure provides confidence and direction, while still allowing flexibility to tailor sessions to each client's needs. Our trainings ensure you master these fundamentals so you can deliver powerful, results-driven sessions.

By asking the right questions, listening closely to your clients and following the 8 steps, you will quickly become skilled at uncovering root causes, building rapport and facilitating transformation through hypnosis.

Chapter 10:

Pre-Talk and Suggestibility Tests

The Power of the Pre-Talk

The success of a hypnosis session often depends on the quality and clarity of the Pre-Talk — the conversation you have with your client before inducing trance. A strong Pre-Talk builds trust, removes misconceptions and creates excitement about the process. When the client feels relaxed, safe and confident that hypnosis will work, they are far more receptive to the session's suggestions.

Addressing Misconceptions

The Pre-Talk is your opportunity to dispel common myths and misconceptions about hypnosis. Many clients arrive with ideas they've picked up from movies or television, or from misconceptions passed down through generations. Here are the most common misconceptions and how you can address them:

I'm going to be 'out' or unconscious

Explain that hypnosis is not about being unconscious or unaware. Hypnosis is a **natural state of focused attention**, like daydreaming or being absorbed in a good book. Most clients will feel calm, relaxed and aware during trance.

You may say, *"Hypnosis feels very familiar because you already enter trance states naturally throughout your day, like when you're driving and miss an exit, or get lost in a good movie or book."*

You'll have control over me

Clarify that all hypnosis is self-hypnosis. The hypnotherapist is simply a guide or facilitator, helping the client achieve their goals. The client remains in complete control and can accept or reject any suggestions at any time.

Try saying, *"Hypnosis is like a dance. I can guide you, but you are always leading yourself. You won't do anything that doesn't align with your values or beliefs."*

What if I get stuck in trance?

Reassure clients that it is impossible to get stuck in trance. Trance is a temporary state, and clients can come out of it naturally or with a simple suggestion.

You could say, *"If I left you in trance, you would simply drift into a restful nap and awaken refreshed and alert. Your mind is always looking after you."*

Addressing these concerns during the Pre-Talk builds confidence and rapport, ensuring that clients are ready to experience a successful session.

Helping the Client Understand the Benefits of Trance

During the Pre-Talk, emphasise the benefits of hypnosis and the role the client plays in their success. Hypnosis works by opening communication with the Unconscious Mind to resolve problems, create new behaviours and activate the body's natural ability to heal.

You may say, *"Trance allows us to plant positive seeds of suggestion in your Unconscious Mind. These suggestions will grow stronger each day, like well-nurtured plants in a fertile garden."*

Explain that hypnosis is a cooperative process. The hypnotherapist provides the guidance, and the client's Unconscious Mind does the work. The more open and receptive the client is, the more effective the session will be.

Suggestibility Tests

Suggestibility tests are an essential part of the Pre-Talk. Their purpose is to demonstrate the power of suggestion, build confidence in the client's ability to respond to hypnosis and help you gauge the client's suggestibility level. These are our recommended beginner-friendly tests:

- **The Bucket and Balloon Test**

Instructions: Ask the client to hold both arms straight out in front of them, palms facing down.

Say: *"Now close your eyes and make a gentle fist with each hand. Imagine that in your left hand, you're holding the handle of a big bucket filled with heavy, wet sand. It's really heavy. You can feel the weight of the bucket of sand pulling your arm downward heavier … and heavier …and heavier … almost like your left arm is being pulled downward by the weight ... down ... down ... down. Now ... in your right hand, imagine a big, bright bunch of helium balloons tied to your right wrist. Helium balloons float, so light that they begin to lift your right arm upward, gently, naturally, effortlessly, lifting your right hand higher and higher. The more you use the power of your intelligence, the power of your imagination, the heavier the bucket becomes, heavier and heavier, and your right hand is being pulled up higher and higher, feeling lighter than air with the balloons lifting ... lifting ... lifting your arm effortlessly. That's right. Now open your eyes."*

Result: When the client opens their eyes, they'll often find their arms have moved, proving the power of suggestion.

- **The Magnetic Fingers Test**

Instructions: Ask the client to clasp their hands together, bend their elbows and extend their two index fingers about two centimetres apart.

Say: *"Imagine there are powerful magnets on the tips of your fingers, pulling them closer and closer together. The harder you try to resist, the stronger the magnetic pull becomes. Closer and closer, closer and closer being pulled faster and faster …"*

Result: Most clients will find their fingers moving closer together involuntarily, showing the influence of their imagination.

- **The Finger Vice Test**

Instructions: Ask the client to clasp their hands together tightly, bend their elbows and raise their index fingers about two centimetres apart.

Say: *"Imagine there is a vice squeezing your fingers tighter and tighter together. Tighter and tighter ... The more you try to resist, the stronger the vice becomes, pulling your fingers together. And when they touch, they will be stuck tight ... the more you try to pull them apart ... the tighter stuck they become. That's right! Now, on the count of three, you can let the vice go and gently separate your fingers ...1, 2, 3.*

Result: *The client will find that their fingers come together and stick tight if you give enough suggestion for that to happen.*

The Body Rotation Test

Instructions: Have the client stand with feet hip-width apart, arms at their sides.

Say: *"Please raise your right arm, point your index finger straight ahead and turn your body to the right as far as you can without moving your feet. Take a mental note of how far you've turned. Now return to the starting position and close your eyes."*

Add *"Now, with your eyes closed, imagine doing it again ... but this time, imagine yourself or see yourself turning much farther — so far that you nearly spin all the way around, as if your body can move freely and effortlessly. That's right, nearly all the way around. Good, now open your eyes."*

Finally: *"Now, please raise your right arm again, point your index finger and turn your body to the right ..."*

Result: Once the client opens their eyes and tries again, they will almost always turn farther than the first time, proving that their Unconscious Mind removes the limits imposed by their Conscious Mind.

Suggestibility Tests as Convincers

These suggestibility tests serve two main purposes:

1. They demonstrate the client's suggestibility. Clients experience firsthand how powerful their imagination and Unconscious Mind can be.

2. They build confidence and trust. The client begins to believe in the process and feels excited to explore the full experience of hypnosis.

For best results, choose 1-3 tests and explain their purpose beforehand. For example, you might say, *"These fun exercises will show you how your mind and body can work together through the power of suggestion and your imagination. Once you see how easy it is, you'll know your mind can achieve great things today."*

If a test doesn't work for a particular client, reassure them that it's perfectly fine — everyone responds differently. Change your wording to better suit your client and remind them to use the power of their intelligence, the power of their imagination and the power of their concentration. Keep the session light, supportive, and encouraging.

Bringing It All Together

The Pre-Talk sets the tone for a successful session by building trust, clarifying misconceptions and creating excitement. By combining an effective Pre-Talk with suggestibility tests like the Bucket/Balloon Test, Magnetic Fingers Test, Finger Vice Test and Arm Rotation Test, you will:

- help your clients feel confident and receptive to the hypnotic process

- demonstrate the power of their imagination and Unconscious Mind

- set the foundation for a smooth, effective trance induction.

Taking the time to get this step right is essential to ensure your clients feel safe, relaxed, understood and ready for transformation. By mastering these techniques, you are creating an environment of trust, confidence and collaboration where life-changing results can occur.

Chapter 11:

Stages of Hypnosis

Understanding Levels of Trance

In order to create successful and impactful hypnotherapy sessions, it is essential to recognise and understand the different levels of hypnosis. As a hypnotherapist, your ability to observe the signs of trance and guide your client through these stages will ensure a smooth, comfortable and beneficial experience.

Recognising levels of trance allows you to:

- utilise what is happening naturally for the client

- deepen the hypnotic state appropriately to achieve your desired outcome

- head off distress by reassuring the client and keeping the process collaborative and relaxed.

Why Recognising Levels of Trance Matters

Each client will respond to hypnosis in their own way, and their ability to reach deeper levels of trance may vary depending on their receptiveness, suggestibility and level of comfort. As you observe the physiological and behavioural cues that indicate trance depth, you can respond in real time, using utilisation techniques (as discussed in Chapter 18) to deepen the trance or reinforce the client's progress.

Failing to recognise the level of trance can sometimes cause unnecessary distress. For example, if a client becomes so relaxed they cannot move their arm, they might panic unless you acknowledge and normalise the experience: *"You may notice now that your arm feels so wonderfully heavy and relaxed that you just don't feel like moving it … and that's perfect. It simply means you're in a deep and comfortable trance."*

By guiding the client confidently and reassuringly through each level, you help them feel safe, relaxed and open to the work you are doing together.

Stages of Hypnosis

The following table outlines the six primary stages of hypnosis and the hypnotic phenomena typically associated with each level. This continuum, provides a useful guide for recognising and utilising trance states effectively.

Stage	Signs & Phenomena	Description
1	Relaxation, Lethargy- Eye Catalepsy	Light trance: Initial relaxation begins. Eyelid catalepsy (unable to open eyes) is common and acts as a strong convincer.
2	Arm/Isolated Muscle Catalepsy- Heavy/ Floating Feelings	Deeper relaxation and catalepsy of small or complete muscle groups, signaling progress to medium trance.
3	Hypnotic Rapport- Smell/Taste Changes- Number Block	Medium trance: Client responds only to the Hypnotherapist, blocking external distractions. Smell/ taste changes and number blocking are possible.
4	Amnesia- Analgesia (No Pain)- Automatic Movement	Deeper medium trance: Client can experience memory gaps, absence of pain (analgesia), and automatic hand or body movements.
5	Positive Hallucinations- Bizarre Post-Hypnotic Suggestions	Deep trance: Client can hallucinate things that do not exist (e.g., seeing or hearing imaginary objects) and respond to creative post-hypnotic suggestions.
6	Negative Hallucinations- Anesthesia (No Feeling)- Somnambulism	Profound trance: Client may not see/hear real stimuli (negative hallucination) and can achieve complete anesthesia. Somnambulism (very deep trance depth) is also possible.

Moving Through the Stages of Hypnosis

Stage 1: Relaxation and Eye Catalepsy

When you first induce trance, clients typically start at Stage 1 with basic relaxation. A hallmark of this stage is eye catalepsy: *"Allow your eyelids to become so relaxed now that the muscles simply won't work ... and when you know they're stuck, you can try to open them and find that they're just too heavy to move."*

This provides a convincing demonstration of light trance and sets the foundation for deeper work.

Stage 2: Arm Catalepsy and Heavy/Floating Feelings

As the trance deepens, isolated muscles or entire muscle groups may experience catalepsy and may also report sensations of heaviness or floating. In these cases, say something like: *"Notice how your arm feels light as a feather ... it may even begin to float upward on its own ... or perhaps it feels so wonderfully heavy, as though it's sinking into the chair."*

These phenomena indicate a progression into medium trance.

Stage 3: Hypnotic Rapport and Sensory Changes

At this stage, you establish hypnotic rapport, where the client's focus is completely on your voice. You can begin eliciting more advanced responses, such as sensory changes (smell, taste) or number blocks.

You can tell your clients, *"As you relax more deeply, you might notice that the fresh cookies I'm holding suddenly smell like sour cabbage ... or perhaps that funny smell just disappears completely."*

And for clients who are experiencing number blocks, you may say, *"The number four has simply vanished. When you count, you'll notice it's no longer there: one, two, three ... five, six ... and it's gone, isn't it?"*

Stage 4: Amnesia, Analgesia, and Automatic Movement

In Stage 4, the client begins experiencing deeper trance phenomena, such as amnesia (forgetting parts of the trance experience) and analgesia (absence of pain). In the latter case, you may say, "You can allow your hand to become completely numb now, as though you're wearing a glove of anesthesia … so relaxed, you wouldn't even feel a pinch or a touch."

Clients' hands or limbs may move without conscious effort, such as rotating their hands in small circles upon suggestion. This is known as automatic movement.

Stage 5: Positive Hallucinations and Post-Hypnotic Suggestions

At this deep trance level, you can elicit positive hallucinations, where clients perceive things that do not exist. You may say, *"You can see a bright red ball in my hand. Notice the texture, the colour and even its weight as you hold it."*

Clients will also respond to more creative post-hypnotic suggestions, such as remembering to drink more water or completing a task effortlessly after the session.

Stage 6: Negative Hallucinations, Anesthesia and Somnambulism

In Stage 6, clients can experience complete anesthesia (no feeling) and negative hallucinations, such as not seeing something that is present. In the latter case, you may say, *"In a moment, you'll no longer see anyone in this room but me … it's as if I'm the only person here."*

Clients may also achieve somnambulism, where they can move and respond while deeply hypnotised, almost appearing to sleepwalk.

Practical Application: Progressing Your Clients Through Trance

1. Observe the signs: Watch for subtle changes in the client's breathing, posture and responses.

2. Utilise what happens: Acknowledge and deepen whatever experience arises naturally. Say, for example, "That's right, as your breathing slows, you're going even deeper now … comfortably and naturally."

3. Recognise the phenomena: Use convincers like eye catalepsy and automatic movement to validate the client's trance experience.

4. Adjust as needed: Not all clients will progress through all stages in one session. Some may need more time or multiple inductions to reach a deep trance.

Conclusion

Mastering the stages of hypnosis will empower you to recognise and utilise the natural progression of trance. The art of hypnotherapy lies in your ability to observe, respond and guide your clients seamlessly through these levels, creating profound and lasting change. With practice, you will become confident in your ability to tailor each session to your client's unique experience, whether they achieve light, medium or deep trance.

Chapter 12:

Developing Your Induction Style

One of the most powerful transitions you can make as a hypnotist is shifting from following scripts to trusting your own style.

We encourage our students to deeply embody the principles of hypnosis, rather than just memorising techniques. That starts with owning your style of induction.

Practise Until It Feels Like Breathing

When you begin, it's completely normal to follow scripts word-for-word. I encourage you to practise the Elman Pre-Talk and Induction with a partner repeatedly. Not until you get it right — but until you can't get it wrong.

As you practise, something beautiful happens. You stop reading and you start feeling. You tune in. You become present. That's when the real magic begins.

Comfort is Critical

Make sure your client is physically comfortable. A hard, straight-backed chair may be fine for a quick chat but it won't work for deep trance. If they feel like they could slide or fall, part of their Unconscious Mind will stay alert and guarded.

Ideally, invest in a comfortable armchair or recliner for your sessions. When a client's body feels supported, their mind relaxes more easily.

Rapport is the First Induction

Rapport is not just about being nice; it's about responsiveness. It's the ability to match someone's world so well that their Unconscious Mind says, "Yes. This person gets me."

Start by matching posture, breathing and subtle movements. If they cross their legs, cross yours. If they lean slightly, match that angle. If their breath is shallow and quick, let your own breath subtly mirror theirs.

It builds trust on an unconscious level.

When you match the breathing rhythm of your client, the entire induction smoothly transitions into a trance-like dance state.

A hypnotist in rapport becomes an extension of the client's experience. They feel guided, not directed.

The Magic of Breathing

One of the most elegant techniques you can use is to match the client's breathing. Speak while they breathe out. Pause when they breathe in. It may interrupt your sentence but that's okay. That rhythm is the induction.

If you're struggling to notice their breath, shift your gaze. Instead of looking directly at them, sit at a 90-degree angle. Let your peripheral vision pick up the movement of their chest. Peripheral vision is naturally tuned to notice motion.

Or, simply listen. Breath makes sound. You can hear their inhale or their sigh, or even notice it when they speak because we speak on the exhale.

Physiology Is Feedback

As you observe your client, remember this: the body doesn't lie.

Every muscle, every twitch, every breath gives you feedback. If the shoulders are relaxed but the neck is tense, you might suggest: *"That's right … and now even the neck can soften and let go."*

If the eyelids begin to flutter, you're witnessing light trance. If the face becomes more symmetrical and the breathing slows, you're deepening.

Learn to read the body as a guide to the mind.

Let Your Voice Follow Them

As the client begins to relax and their head tilts forward, gently lower your own head as well. Your voice should follow their descent. By the time you reach the number steps of the Elman Induction, you may be speaking directly to their knees or feet.

This directional change affects the Unconscious Mind. It signals safety, depth and progression. It also anchors trance through spatial association.

Invite Feedback

Sometimes, the best way to grow is simply to ask.

After a full induction, including suggestions and a re-induction anchor, bring your client back and ask: *"How was that for you?"*

You'll get valuable insights about pacing, timing and which suggestions resonated. Then, when you guide them back into trance, you can tailor your approach even more precisely.

Let Intuition Take the Lead

As your confidence grows, allow your Unconscious Mind to participate in the session. Be open to spontaneous language or using what the client presents. One day, you might find yourself saying something like: *"And as soon as your mind is clear and open, you might find a finger lifting, letting me know you're ready."* And the client will lift their finger as if they knew all along.

This is utilisation. This is responsiveness. This is real hypnosis.

The Waking Trance

Great hypnotists often find themselves entering a waking trance alongside their client. Milton Erickson referred to it often. When you're truly connected, it feels like time slows down. Words come from somewhere deeper. You stop doing hypnosis and start being hypnotic.

When you're in rapport, when you're observing keenly and when you're present with your client transformation unfolds with ease.

Final Thought

Your induction style is yours to create. Start with structure. Practise it until it lives in your bones. Then let it evolve. Let it become art.

When you trust yourself and deeply tune in to your client, you become the induction.

Chapter 13:

The Elman Method – Fast, Deep, Reliable Hypnosis

I f Milton Erickson was the master of elegant, indirect language, then Dave Elman was the no-nonsense engineer of deep trance.

Elman's approach is fast, structured and direct. It works beautifully when you want to bypass the Critical Faculty swiftly and lead your client into a responsive, powerful state for change.

Dave Elman was one of the great pioneers of medical hypnosis. His work is so practical and so effective that many of the rapid induction techniques still used by doctors, dentists and hypnotherapists around the world come directly from him. He understood that hypnosis isn't something you do to someone but something they do for themselves.

In 1964, Elman[1] famously wrote: *"There is really no such thing as a hypnotist ... You won't hypnotize them; they will hypnotize themselves."*

What I love most about Elman's approach is that it's accessible. It's built on the beautiful principle that all hypnosis is self-hypnosis. That means you're not 'doing' something to a client; you're showing them how to access a powerful state within themselves. Elman made hypnosis feel safe, simple and natural — for practitioner and client alike.

---

1. Elman, D., (1964) *Hypnotherapy*, Westwood Publishing Co

In this chapter, we're going to explore exactly how Elman's methods work, why they're so effective and how to use them confidently with your own clients.

Who was Dave Elman?

Dave Elman wasn't a doctor or a psychologist. He actually started his career in entertainment and radio, but don't let that fool you because he had an extraordinary ability to simplify what others had overcomplicated. Elman's father had used hypnosis to relieve pain when he was dying from cancer, and that experience stayed with Elman for life.

Eventually, Elman began teaching hypnosis to doctors and dentists at the request of the American Medical Association. Published in 1964, his book, *Hypnotherapy*, is a collection of real-world cases and practical techniques that have stood the test of time.

Elman wasn't interested in theories that didn't get results. He was deeply focused on what worked — and how fast. That's why his methods remain at the heart of our clinical hypnosis training today.

Why Learn the Elman Method?

There are many ways to guide someone into trance. Some are indirect and permissive (like Erickson's methods) and some are authoritarian and direct (like traditional hypnosis). Elman's genius was that his method could be both. He knew how to:

- bypass the critical mind quickly

- set up dissociation between the conscious and unconscious

- achieve deep trance with structure and flow.

His background in stage hypnosis and clinical work with doctors gave Elman the perfect balance of speed and depth. He needed a way to hypnotise someone deeply in minutes, and he created it.

One of the reasons we love teaching the Elman Induction is that it isn't just fast and reliable — it's elegant. And it places full ownership in the hands of the client, where all real transformation lives.

Elman's Hypnotic Philosophy: Simplicity and Speed

Elman believed that hypnosis was a natural state that anyone could access quickly, safely and deeply, with the right guidance. His inductions are direct and efficient. No fluff. No unnecessary confusion.

Let's look at a few of Elman's core beliefs that shape how we teach and practice.

- Hypnosis is not sleep: although it may look like sleep to an outsider, the client remains aware and alert.

- Depth matters: Elman was one of the first to clearly articulate the importance of reaching somnambulism (a deep trance state) for therapeutic work.

- Hypnosis is a learning state: The client learns how to go into trance, how to respond to suggestions and how to shift their internal experience.

Now, let's dive into the method itself.

What Makes the Elman Method Different?

The following table shows how Elman's approach fits into the bigger picture:

Type of Hypnosis	Client Approach	Induction Style	Trance Type
Traditional hypnosis	Authoritarian	Direct	Sleeping
Erickson hypnosis	Permissive	Indirect	Waking or sleeping
NLP	Authoritarian	Indirect	Waking
Elman hypnosis	Authoritarian or permissive	Direct or indirect	Waking or sleeping

Elman wasn't locked into one style. That means you can tailor the Elman Induction to suit the client in front of you and whether they prefer structure, flow, fast pace or gentle guidance.

But his greatest innovation? The use of paradox and selective thinking: close your eyes and pretend you can't open them ... knowing full well that you can.

This playful use of paradox confuses the Critical Faculty just enough to let the Unconscious begin accepting suggestion. The client is invited into a trance process in which their own imagination does the work. When they 'test' the suggestion and find that their eyes won't open, they immediately experience a form of truth that goes beyond logic. This is powerful. This is hypnotic.

Another of Elman's core principles is: selective thinking is what you believe wholeheartedly.

If the client believes, even temporarily, that something is true (e.g. "I can't open my eyes"), that selective thinking becomes the entry point into trance. The moment doubt creeps in, trance fades. The moment belief strengthens, trance deepens.

How to Deliver an Elman Induction

Before you ever begin the induction, you must do what Elman considered essential: the Pre-Talk.

This is more than a warm-up. It sets the psychological conditions required for hypnosis to occur. Without it, you may find yourself meeting resistance, confusion or doubt.

Elman's Four Preconditions for Hypnosis

1. Consent: the client must agree to be hypnotised.

2. Communication: there must be rapport and clear understanding.

3. Freedom from fear: the client must feel emotionally safe.

4. Trust: the client must trust you and the process.

If any of these are missing, the induction will stall.

Elman Pre-Talk

"Let me show you something interesting. Make a tight fist with your hand. Now relax it."

We know we can tense a muscle until it can't go any tighter. We also know we can relax a muscle so completely that unless we choose to change it, it simply won't work.

The easiest muscles to do this with are our eyelids. Think of how good it feels to close your eyes when you're tired. It's soft, heavy and comfortable. So, try this with your clients:

"Watch me. I'm going to relax my eyes so fully, that unless I choose to remove that relaxation, they won't work." (Demonstrate.) "Now I'll try to open them, and see? Nothing. I could open them if I really wanted to. But I don't. I'm simply holding on to the suggestion. Now it's your turn. Close your eyes and relax those muscles. Pretend you can't open them. Really pretend. Test them. That's right ... Congratulations. That's the first step. You just created a hypnotic effect — yourself."

This is a key message to embed: you are not hypnotising the client. The client is hypnotising themselves with your guidance.

Elman Induction #1 (Step-by-Step)

1. Deep Breath and Eye Closure

"Take a long deep breath ... and as you exhale, let your eyes gently close."

2. Eye Catalepsy (Tested Suggestion)

"Place your awareness on your eye muscles. Let those muscles go soft ... completely relaxed ... to the point they just won't work. When you're sure they're so relaxed that they won't work unless you choose to make them work, hold on to that feeling and test them. Try to open them while holding onto the relaxation. Test them hard. That's right."

3. Flowing Relaxation Through the Body

"Now, let that same relaxation flow from the top of your head all the way down your body ... like a warm wave ... past your shoulders, down your arms, through your chest, your hips, your legs ... all the way to your toes."

4. Fractionation

Fractionation is a classic hypnotic technique where the client is guided to move in and out of trance repeatedly. Each time they 'come up' and then 'go back down', the depth of trance increases. Think of it like working a muscle; with each repetition, the Unconscious learns how to drop into trance more quickly and more deeply.

It works because contrast strengthens the experience. By briefly returning the client to a lighter state and then back into trance, the difference makes the depth feel more profound. This is why Elman's Induction is both fast and reliable. Fractionation deepens trance in just a few cycles.

"In a moment, I'll ask you to open and close your eyes again. When you close them, allow yourself to go ten times deeper into this feeling. Ready? Open your eyes … and now close your eyes … going ten times deeper. We'll do this again. Open your eyes … and close them … doubling that depth. That's right."

(Repeat until client is visibly showing trance signs: facial flushing, slower breathing, stillness, minimal blink rate.)

5. Arm Drop Test (Physical Suggestibility)

"I'm going to gently lift your hand. Don't help me. Let it be heavy and loose like a wet dishrag. When I let go, just let it drop and feel yourself going deeper."

(Lift wrist a few inches and drop it. If the arm flops, proceed. If not, say "Don't help me" and try again.)

6. Mental Relaxation (Number Block)

"Now, to relax your mind as deeply as your body, we'll use numbers. I want you to begin counting backwards slowly from 100 out loud. With each number, double your mental relaxation. Let the numbers begin to fade. By the time you reach 98, or even sooner, they might disappear completely. Begin now. 100 … (pause) 99 … (pause) 98 … fading. Are they all gone? Good."

This is somnambulism — the ideal state for therapy, suggestion work and transformation.

The Second Elman Induction (Faster Version)

Once a client has experienced the first induction, the second version moves much faster. The steps are the same but with tighter pacing. This is especially useful for repeat sessions or clients who go into trance easily.

1. Deep Breath & Eye Closure

"Take a deep breath. And as you exhale, close your eyes."

2. Eye Catalepsy (Brief Version)

"Relax the muscles around your eyes so completely they just won't work. Pretend they can't open, even though you know they can. Hold onto that, and test them. That's it."

3. Body Relaxation

"Let that same quality of deep relaxation move through your whole body now ... effortlessly."

4. Fractionation Quickening

"Open your eyes. Close your eyes. Double the relaxation. Open your eyes. Close your eyes. Again, double the depth."

5. Arm Drop

"I'll lift your arm and drop it. Let it flop. Let that deepen your trance."

6. Number Block Fast

"Begin counting from 100 backwards. With each number, relax more. Let the numbers start to fade ... 100 ... 99 ... 98 ... gone. Are they all gone? That's right."

The Four Levels of Trance

According to Elman, there are four levels of trance:

1. Light Trance (Eye Catalepsy) – the starting place.

2. Physical Relaxation – body unresponsive, loose, limp.

3. Mental Relaxation / Somnambulism – the Critical Faculty is bypassed.

4. Coma State (Esdaile) – rare and profound; the mind becomes 'blank', like the moment before falling asleep.

What If You Master This?

When you master the Elman method, you'll have a go-to induction that works quickly, reliably and beautifully in a wide range of contexts. You'll also understand how to tailor your hypnotic work to the client in front of you — whether they need something structured, permissive, fast or slow.

This method is a cornerstone of your skillset. Practise it. Memorise the flow. Feel into the timing. And most importantly — make it your own.

As Dave Elman himself said: "There is nothing I can do that you can't learn to do in hypnosis."

That's true. And now it's your turn.

Chapter 14:

Ericksonian Methods

The Power of Erickson's Indirect Techniques

Having a broad range of hypnotic techniques allows you to adapt to any client. Among the most influential contributions to modern hypnotherapy are **Milton Erickson's indirect and permissive techniques**, which forever changed the way hypnosis is practised.

Erickson's brilliance lay in his ability to move away from the older, authoritarian styles of hypnosis. Instead of saying, "Close your eyes and relax," Erickson would seamlessly weave his suggestions into natural conversations, bypassing the client's Conscious Mind and speaking directly to their Unconscious Mind. By the time the client left the session, changes had begun, often without them consciously realising how it happened.

Erickson's methods are particularly valuable for clients or individuals who:

- are uncomfortable with direct suggestions or authority-based approaches

- may be skeptical of hypnosis or trying it for the first time

- need a gentle, permissive induction tailored to their comfort and receptiveness.

Whether you work with direct techniques (like Elman Inductions) or indirect techniques (like Ericksonian methods), knowing both styles makes you a versatile and effective hypnotherapist. Erickson's methods are also foundational for anyone studying NLP and will be explored deeply in the NLP Practitioner and Master Practitioner trainings.

Erickson's Utilisation Approach

One of Erickson's most profound ideas was utilisation: the ability to use everything the client says, does or experiences as part of the hypnosis process. Erickson recognised that every client has a unique 'model of the world' – their personal beliefs, values and experiences that influence how they think, feel and behave. To help clients change, he would first loosen their current model of the world so they could open themselves to new ideas and solutions.

Erickson's utilisation approach can be broken into three key stages:

1. Preparation – establishing rapport, identifying the client's presenting problem and addressing misconceptions. This was covered in previous chapters (Pre-Talk, Personal History and Suggestibility Tests).

2. Trance Work – inducing trance using indirect, permissive techniques. This is the core hypnosis session, where Erickson's methods come to life.

3. Evaluation of Results – ensuring the client acknowledges the changes made during trance, reinforcing success. A joint review by the hypnotherapist and client that solidifies the positive changes made.

Steps for Ericksonian Trance Work

1. Fixation of Attention

Rather than using traditional fixation objects like a swinging pendulum, Erickson focused the client's attention on their inner experience: "I wonder if you've noticed how comfortable you're feeling as you sit here ... *listening to my voice ... and beginning to become aware of your breathing ... that natural, easy rhythm.*"

This indirect focus naturally begins to draw the client into trance.

2. Loosening the Client's Model of the World

To make deep change possible, you need to help clients shift their limiting beliefs or assumptions. Questions from the 'Keys to an Achievable Outcome' (taught in NLP Practitioner Training) can prepare them for change: *"What do you want? What will achieving this allow you to do? What resources do you already have, or need, to make this happen?"*

By bringing the client's focus to new possibilities, you begin to plant the seeds of transformation.

3. Ericksonian Patterns of Indirect Suggestion

Erickson's hypnotic techniques include a variety of subtle, effective patterns that bypass resistance and engage the Unconscious Mind.

Let's explore these techniques with practical examples you can start using immediately.

Ericksonian Hypnotic Patterns

- **Indirect Suggestions**

Indirect suggestions avoid direct commands and are less likely to trigger resistance. They bypass the Critical Faculty by phrasing commands in a softer, conversational manner. Instead of saying, "Close your eyes" (direct), you might say, "You might begin to wonder how it feels to simply let your eyes close … when you're ready" (indirect).

This phrasing sounds more like curiosity than a command, encouraging the Unconscious Mind to respond naturally.

- **Embedded Commands**

Embedded commands are instructions hidden within a larger sentence. They allow you to give suggestions that the client's Unconscious Mind hears and follows without triggering conscious evaluation.

For example:

- *"You might not realise just yet how deeply you can relax … but you can begin to relax … now."*

- *"As you listen to my voice, you may find that you go into trance comfortably and easily."*

Tip: pausing slightly or changing your tone when saying the embedded command can make it even more effective.

The embedded command is *"relax ... now"* and *"go into trance"*. The Unconscious Mind hears these, even as the Conscious Mind focuses on the rest of the sentence.

- **Embedded Descriptions**

Embedded descriptions describe experiences as if they are hypothetical, but the Unconscious Mind hears them as real possibilities. For instance: "Some people find that as they listen to the sound of my voice, they begin to drift into a comfortable, relaxed state."

This phrasing allows the client to unconsciously accept the suggestion of relaxation without feeling pressured.

- **Truisms about Sensations**

Truisms are statements that are obviously true and help guide the client into trance by building agreement.

For example:

"Most people find that focusing on their breathing helps them relax."

"You may notice how one of your hands feel slightly warmer or heavier than the other now ... "

Pairing truisms with sensory focus deepens trance naturally.

- **Truisms Utilising Time**

Time-related suggestions imply that something will naturally happen, leaving the timing up to the client. This allows the Unconscious Mind to accept the suggestion comfortably.

For example:

- *"In a moment, you might notice your eyelids feeling heavier."*

- *"Sooner or later, you may find your mind drifting to a calm, peaceful place."*

These suggestions build anticipation and pave the way for deeper trance.

Not Knowing, Not Doing

This technique uses paradoxical language to suggest that the client doesn't need to actively 'try'. Instead, the process happens naturally.

For example:

- *"You don't have to know how to relax … it just happens all by itself."*

- *"You may not know exactly when your breathing slows … and that's perfectly fine."*

- *"You don't have to talk or move or make any sort of effort."*

- *"You don't even have to hold your eyes open."*

By taking the pressure off, the Unconscious Mind becomes more open to following the suggestion.

- **Open-Ended Suggestions**

Open-ended suggestions invite the client's Unconscious Mind to find the best solutions for them.

For example:

- *"I wonder what positive changes your mind will discover for you today … and how you will use them in your life."*

- *"You might notice how you're already beginning to feel better, in a way that's perfect for you."*

- *"I'm curious if you'll feel that relaxation in your shoulders or your arms first."*

- *"We all have potential we are unaware of and we usually don't know how it will be expressed."*

This approach respects the client's autonomy while engaging their Unconscious Mind.

Covering All Possible Responses

This technique ensures that no matter what happens, the suggestion applies. It removes pressure and increases acceptance.

For example:

- *"Your arm might feel heavy ... or light ... or it might not move at all — and that's perfectly fine."*

- *"Tonight when you sleep you may dream. You may have wild dreams ... you may have exciting dreams ... you may have mild dreams ... you may have boring dreams. Your dreams may be memorable or they may not. In any case, let that be a sign ... that you are integrating everything at the Unconscious level. So that by this time tomorrow, you will know everything you need to know in order to have the problem disappear."*

Whatever the client experiences is framed as the correct response, reinforcing their sense of success.

Questions to Facilitate Change

Erickson often used questions to focus the client's attention inward and promote change.

For example:

- *"I wonder how quickly you'll begin to notice the changes happening inside you?"*

- *"Have you ever noticed how much easier things can feel when you let go of old habits?*

- *"Did you experience the hypnotic state as basically similar to the waking state or different from the waking state?*

Questions bypass resistance by creating curiosity and engaging the Unconscious Mind.

Compound Suggestions

Compound suggestions combine multiple linguistic or psychological elements into a single suggestion. They make the Unconscious Mind more likely to accept and act upon the message because they bypass resistance, link ideas and offer multiple entry points for influence. Think of them as 'multi-layered messages' — one suggestion piggybacks on another, or unfolds in steps, so the client's unconscious finds it easier to say yes.

Here are the main types, with added explanation and examples:

a. Yes Set

A Yes Set is a series of undeniable statements that build agreement and rapport. Once the client is saying or thinking 'yes,' they are more likely to agree to a deeper suggestion.

For example:

- *"You are sitting here ... listening to my voice ... breathing naturally ... and noticing how easy it is to relax in the comfort of the chair."*

- *"It is such a beautiful day, the sun is shining, and you are sitting here comfortably ... so it makes sense to just let your mind drift even more easily."*

By stacking a series of 'yes' responses, the client becomes naturally receptive to deeper suggestions.

Start with undeniable truths, then slip in the suggestion.

b. Associations

This form links the client's natural processes (breathing, blinking, sensations) to the desired response. The association makes the suggestion feel inevitable and natural.

For example: *"With each breath you take, you can become more aware of the natural rhythms of your body ... and those rhythms allow feelings of calm to deepen."*

Tie the suggestion to something the client is already doing automatically.

c. Opposites

By contrasting two experiences, opposites create balance and a sense of inevitability. The Unconscious looks for harmony between the two.

For example: *"As one hand becomes lighter, the other may press down more heavily."*

Use the natural tendency to compare and balance opposites to reinforce trance.

d. Negative – Tag Questions

These appear to invite doubt but actually presuppose agreement. The 'tag' hooks the unconscious into a 'yes'.

For example:

- *"And you can, can you not?"*

- *"You can try, can't you?"*

- *"You can't stop it, can you?"*

Tag questions soften the suggestion, making it feel less like an order and more like a choice.

e. Negative – Until

These suggestions cleverly delay the desired response, giving the Unconscious permission to wait, which, ironically, sets it up to respond.

For example:

- *"You don't have to go into trance until you're ready."*

- *"You won't do it until your unconscious is ready."*

Resistance drops because the Unconscious hears, "You don't have to yet", which lowers pressure and makes the change easier.

f. Shock or Surprise

These suggestions interrupt the client's usual patterns, creating an opening for the Unconscious to accept a new idea.

Suggestions include:

- **Abrupt pauses and breaks in rhythm**

"Your life … (pause) … just what you need to know about it … (pause) … secretly what you want … (pause) … is more important now."

The pause or unexpected twist captures attention, destabilises conscious resistance and drops the suggestion into the Unconscious.

- **Unexpected contrasts**

"Some people think change takes years … others discover it can happen in a single breath."

The surprise contrast reframes expectations and opens possibilities.

- **Odd and playful images**

"As you sit there comfortably, listening to my words … a pink elephant might seem silly … and yet that silliness shows how quickly your mind can shift focus."

Unusual images capture attention and create openings for suggestion.

- **Disruption of meaning**

"Your eyes can close now … or later … or maybe they've already closed in your mind, even if they're open."

The Conscious Mind hiccups; the Unconscious accepts the flow.

- **Surprise questions**

"What colour is the thought of calm in your mind right now?"

The mind scrambles to answer, bypassing Critical Filters.

- **Incomplete sentences**

"And as you notice that feeling begin to spread ... you might already ..." (Pause and let their mind complete it.)

The Unconscious rushes to fill the gap with its own suggestion.

Double Binds

Double binds give the illusion of choice while ensuring that both options lead to the desired outcome.

For example:

- *"Would you like to go into trance now, or would you prefer to feel even more relaxed first?"*

- *"You can notice how calm you feel now ... or in a few moments."*

- *"Would you prefer to relax deeply now ... or in just a few moments?"*

- *"You can choose to drift deeper with every breath ... or every word I say."*

The client feels in control, yet the outcome is the same: they enter trance.

Using Erickson's Patterns in Trance Work

The power of Erickson's methods lies in their subtlety. Rather than forcing a trance state, Ericksonian Hypnosis invites the Unconscious Mind to cooperate naturally. For beginners, practise integrating the following:

- Start with Yes Sets to build rapport.

- Add Embedded Commands and Truisms during trance induction.

- Use Open-Ended Suggestions to deepen the experience.

Example of a Simple Induction

1. "You are sitting here, comfortably, listening to my voice." (Yes Set)

2. "And as you take a slow, gentle breath ... you may notice your body relaxing." (Truism About Sensations)

3. "I'm curious if you'll feel that relaxation in your shoulders or your arms first." (Open-Ended Suggestion)

4. "And you don't have to try to make it happen … it just happens all by itself." (Not Knowing, Not Doing)

Evaluating Results: Locking in Change

After trance work, ensure your client acknowledges the change.

For example:

- *" What feels different now?"*

- *"Can you try to find that old feeling … and notice how it's no longer there?"*

If they affirm the change, you've successfully integrated the work. Encourage them to describe their progress in their own words to strengthen their belief in the transformation.

Conclusion

Milton Erickson's methods empower you to guide clients into trance in a way that feels natural, comfortable and deeply effective. By learning to utilise everything the client brings, you will create truly tailored and transformative sessions.

Mastering these indirect techniques gives you the tools to work confidently with clients at all levels. From embedded commands to double binds, Erickson's approach will help you facilitate lasting change and establish yourself as a world-class hypnotherapist.

In the next chapter, we will explore classic Ericksonian inductions, demonstrating how to seamlessly combine these powerful hypnotic patterns in real-world sessions.

Chapter 15:

Two Ericksonian Inductions

In this chapter, we begin the practical application of Ericksonian hypnosis techniques. To become a confident hypnotherapist, it's essential to experience the process both as a client and as a facilitator. The more you practise, the more natural and instinctive these inductions will become.

Start with simple inductions, such as the Question Set Induction and the Arm Levitation Induction described here. These methods are accessible for beginners and are built on Erickson's indirect, permissive style.

Tip for Beginners

Practising with a partner is essential. Choose someone curious, open-minded and willing to explore hypnosis with you. Take turns as the hypnotherapist and client to develop your confidence and understanding.

Ericksonian Induction No. 1: The Question Set Induction

This first induction focuses on eliciting trance through a series of gentle, non-directive questions. It's perfect for new hypnotherapists because it uses natural language and curiosity to guide the client into a relaxed, trance-like state. This induction can take approximately 10-15 minutes.

Step-by-Step Process

1. Have you ever been in a trance before ... right now?

This question naturally draws the client's focus inward. If they say "No," relate the question to a familiar experience:

Ask: Can you remember the last time you were completely absorbed in a book or movie? Can you remember the state you were in just before you woke up this morning?

These questions subtly lead the client to recall everyday trance states.

2. Did you experience that state as being similar to the waking state, or different from it? Asking this question deepens their focus on the experience and nudges them further into trance.

3. Can you find a spot (above eye level) that you would like to look at comfortably?

Direct their gaze to fixate on a point, above, to encourage relaxation. Eye fixation is a classic way to deepen trance.

4. As you comfortably look at that spot, do your eyelids want to blink?

Observe the client's natural blinking pattern. When they blink, say softly, "That's right ..."

This encourages the Unconscious to follow your subtle cues.

5. Will those lids begin to blink one at a time... twice... or three times before they close altogether?

Here you are pacing the client's experience while implying what happens next — closure of the eyes.

6. Rapidly or more slowly?

Keep the tone curious and permissive. The client's mind accepts the suggestion at its own pace.

7. Will they just close now, or flutter all by themselves first?

If eyelids flutter, this indicates a shift deeper into trance. Gently validate this with "That's right."

8. Will your eyes close more and more as you get more and more relaxed?

This reinforces the natural progression into relaxation.

9. That's right. Can those eyes just stay closed as you go deeper ... just like when you go to sleep?

Use a soothing voice here to guide them into a deeper state of calm.

10. Or would you rather try in vain to open them, and find you cannot?

This suggestion adds a light challenge while implying relaxation. Clients often find their eyelids feel heavier.

11. And just when will you forget about your eyes altogether because your Unconscious Mind wants you to dream... now?

The word *dream* can prompt the Unconscious to go deeper into a relaxed, dreamy state.

Insert Suggestions

Once the client is in a relaxed state, provide positive, clear suggestions based on what they want to achieve, repeating the one suggestion in different ways at least three times (see Chapter 17).

For example:

- *"Your Unconscious Mind can integrate everything you're learning and help you become a confident hypnotherapist."*

- *"Each time you practise, you'll naturally find hypnosis becoming easier and more effective."*

Bring the Client Out of Trance

Say gently: "In a moment, I will count backwards from 10 to 1, and you will awaken one tenth of the way with each number until you are fully awake. 10 ... 9 ... 8 ... That's right, returning refreshed ... 7 ... 6 ... and clear-headed ... 5

... 4 ... all the way back to the present ... 3 ... 2 ... and 1. Wide awake now, feeling good and ready to move forward."

What to Observe

As a beginner, note your partner's breathing, blinking and any visible muscle relaxation. These are clear signs of trance. Validate these signs with a simple "That's right." Remember, every small response is a success.

Ericksonian Induction No. 2: Arm Levitation

The Arm Levitation Induction is an excellent example of Milton Erickson's indirect, permissive approach to trance. It uses the client's natural breathing rhythm as a physiological anchor:

- Out-Breath: reinforces relaxation and deepening trance.

- In-Breath: encourages arm movement and levitation.

Your goal is to guide the client into a light or medium trance while eliciting natural hand movement, using pacing, permissive language and subtle embedded suggestions.

Step-by-Step Script with Explanations

1. Begin Relaxation – Speaking on the Out-Breath

Focus on guiding the client into a comfortable state. Use pacing and relaxation suggestions.

a. "Have you ever been in a trance before... right now?" (*Speak softly on the client's out-breath.*)

This question encourages the client to focus internally and consider their experience of trance, a process that naturally deepens relaxation.

b. "Did you experience that state as being similar to the waking state, or different from the waking state?" (*Out-breath*)

This question further draws the client inward, as they reflect on prior trance-like experiences, such as the driving trance or daydreaming.

2. Introduce Arm Levitation – Speaking on the In-Breath

Begin to suggest hand movement, linking it subtly to the inhale. The tone of your voice remains gentle and conversational.

c. "You can feel comfortable resting your hands gently on your thighs, can you not?" *(In-breath)*

Demonstrate a light touch of the fingertips on the thighs. Ensure the client's hands feel relaxed and neutral.

d. "That's right. Don't let them touch each other ... just resting so lightly." *(In-breath)*

This sets up the idea of lightness and primes the suggestion of upward movement.

e. "Can you let those hands rest so-oo lightly ... so that the fingertips just touch your thighs?" *(In-breath)*

Reinforces the feeling of lightness and increases awareness of the hands.

3. Observe and Validate Small Movements – Speaking on the In-Breath

Pay attention to small, natural movements (e.g. a twitch, subtle lift). Acknowledge these to build unconscious responsiveness.

f. "That's right. As they rest there just so lightly ... have you noticed yet how they tend to lift up a bit all by themselves?" *(Take an audible in-breath as you say "lift").*

Your in-breath cues the client's inhale and encourages unconscious arm movement.

g. "With each breath you take ... just a little higher ... all by themselves." *(In-breath)*

Speak gently on the client's inhale, creating rhythm and alignment with their breathing.

h. "Good. Now we'll just wait and see ..." *(Pause after speaking to allow for response.)*

A moment of silence allows the Unconscious Mind to process and respond naturally.

4. Deepen Relaxation If No Movement Occurs – Speaking on the Out-Breath

If the hands have not yet begun to lift, deepen relaxation first.

i. "Now, can you find a spot that you would like to look at comfortably?" *(Out-breath)*

j. "As you continue comfortably looking at that spot for a while, do your eyelids want to blink?" *(Out-breath)*

Guide the client toward eye closure as a signal of deepening trance.

k. "Will those lids begin to blink ... one at a time ... twice or three times before they close altogether?" *(Out-breath)*

l. "Will the eyes close more and more as you get more and more relaxed?" *(Out-breath)*

m. "That's right. Can those eyes just stay closed ... as you're comfortable to go deeper, just like when you go to sleep?" *(Out-breath)*

n. "And can your comfort go more and more deeply inside ... so that you'd rather not even try to open your eyes?" *(Out-breath)*

o. "Or would you rather really try in vain ... and find you cannot?" *(Out-breath)*

These questions deepen relaxation and focus the Unconscious Mind on internal sensations.

5. Resume Arm Levitation – Speaking on the In-Breath

Transition back to eliciting arm movement. Speak gently and match the rhythm of the client's in-breaths.

p. "Have you noticed your hands lifting ... lifting ... lifting ... even more lightly, even more easily ... and by themselves ... as the rest of your body relaxes more and more?" *(In-breath)*

q. "As that goes on, does one hand or the other … or maybe both … continue lifting, lifting, lifting even more?" *(In-breath)*

r. "And does that hand stay up and continue lifting, lifting, lifting even higher and higher all by itself?" *(In-breath)*

s. "Does the other hand want to catch up with it and go up too … or will the other hand just relax in your lap?" *(In-breath)*

t. "Now … does the hand slow down … or go faster and faster as it approaches your face … deepening your comfort?" *(In-breath)*

u. "And will your body automatically take a deeper breath when that hand touches your face … as you really relax and go even deeper?" *(In-breath)*

6. Validate and Transition – Speaking on the Out-Breath

Acknowledge progress and guide the client further into trance.

v. "That's right. And as that hand slowly begins to drift back to your lap … you can notice how that calm, comfortable feeling deepens even more … as your Unconscious Mind integrates everything perfectly." *(Out-breath)*

7. Insert Positive Suggestions

Once arm levitation is complete, deliver desired positive suggestions based on the client's outcome: "And as you relax deeply now … your Unconscious Mind can continue to make those positive changes you came here for, easily and naturally." *(Out-breath)*

8. Bring the Client Out of Trance

Gently bring the client back to full awareness: "In a moment, I'm going to count backwards from 10 to 1. With each number, you'll come back to full awareness, feeling refreshed and calm. 10 … 9 … 8 … becoming more aware … 7 … 6 … 5 … taking a deep breath … 4 … 3 … 2 … and 1 … fully awake now, feeling wonderful."

Key Notes for Beginners

- Aim to speak on the client's in-breath when eliciting arm movement (e.g. "lifting, lifting, lifting").

- Use the out-breath to deepen relaxation and comfort (e.g. "relax more deeply now").

- Keep your tone soft, permissive, and encouraging. Use pauses to allow the client time to respond naturally.

- Always validate progress with "That's right" to reinforce suggestions and build rapport.

With practice, this timing will become second nature, allowing you to guide clients into a smooth and effective Ericksonian trance experience.

Why Use Arm Levitation?

Arm levitation serves as a convincer, showing the client the power of their Unconscious Mind. The physical movement of their arm acts as undeniable proof that hypnosis is working. It also deepens trust in the process.

Summary

These two Ericksonian inductions are simple yet powerful tools for building confidence in your ability as a hypnotherapist. They are effective, comfortable for the client and utilise Erickson's indirect and permissive style.

Practising these inductions repeatedly will help you develop your own rhythm, tonality and phrasing. You will soon notice how effortlessly clients respond to your guidance as you continue on this exciting journey of mastering hypnosis.

Breathing and Tonality Tips for Beginners

1. Speak on the In-Breath for Movement. Suggestions for arm levitation should always align with the client's inhale.

For example:

- *"With each breath in … notice how your hand begins to lift …"*

Take a deep, audible breath yourself as you say words like 'lift' to encourage mirroring.

2. Speak on the Out-Breath for Relaxation. Suggestions for deepening relaxation align with the client's exhale.

For example:

- *"As that hand lifts ... the rest of your body relaxes ... even more deeply."*

3. Pause and Observe. Allow moments of silence after suggestions. This gives the client time to respond naturally.

4. Use "That's Right" for Validation. Whenever you notice small movements, such as a slight twitch or lift, acknowledge it softly:

- *"That's right ... just letting it happen ... easily and naturally."*

Why It Works

The Arm Levitation Induction is an Ericksonian classic because it utilises natural processes (like breathing and muscle relaxation) to bypass the Critical Faculty. By aligning suggestions with the client's natural rhythm, the Unconscious Mind takes over, allowing effortless movement and deep relaxation.

Remember, the movement does not have to be dramatic. Even a slight lift is a success because it demonstrates the Unconscious Mind's response to suggestion.

With practice, coordinating your timing with the client's breathing will feel natural. Soon, you'll find yourself confidently guiding clients into a deep, peaceful trance using this elegant and effective Ericksonian induction.

Key Notes for Timing

1. Out-Breath: Use this to suggest relaxation, eye closure and deepening of trance.

2. In-Breath: Use this to encourage hand movement and lightness.

3. Breathing Cue: Breathe audibly to synchronise with the client and pause to allow time for their Unconscious Mind to respond.

4. Reinforcement: Always validate progress with "That's right" to build trust and rapport with the Unconscious Mind.

Chapter 16:

The Progressive Test Induction — Blending Styles for Deep Trance Mastery

Throughout your training so far, you've learned how powerful permissive, indirect approaches to hypnosis can be — particularly for helping clients relax, build rapport and enter a receptive state of mind.

Now, you're ready to take the next step: learning a method that combines both the permissive style of Milton Erickson and the direct, authoritarian style pioneered by earlier hypnotists like George Estabrooks.

This method is called the Progressive Test Induction, and it will quickly become one of the most useful tools in your hypnotherapy toolkit.

Why Learn the Progressive Test Induction?

The Progressive Test Induction is a beautifully structured process that allows clients to experience progressively deeper states of trance through simple, natural tests — such as feeling their eyelids lock shut, or discovering their arms move automatically.

Each 'test' acts as a:

- convincer (showing the client their unconscious mind is responding)

- deepener (taking them deeper into hypnosis naturally)

- builder of unconscious skill (leading to greater success later)

It's a fun, safe and effective way to guide someone from light relaxation into a profound hypnotic state — even if they've never experienced trance before.

As a hypnotist, you'll love it because it:

- gives you visible phenomena you can use to confirm depth

- allows natural progression without needing to force anything

- blends Ericksonian utilisation with direct suggestion beautifully

- teaches your client (and their unconscious mind) how to be hypnotised with growing confidence.

Where the Progressive Test Induction Came From

The original seeds of this induction were planted in the work of George Estabrooks, a professor and hypnosis expert who published Hypnosis in 1943 and Hypnotism in 1946. Across both texts, Estabrooks outlined a highly structured, authoritative approach to hypnosis designed to produce deep trance phenomena quickly and reliably.

His methods were especially effective for producing clear hypnotic phenomena and post-hypnotic responses, where conscious interference diminished and the unconscious mind could operate more freely.

Decades later, Tad James adapted and expanded this approach, combining Estabrooks' structure with Ericksonian language patterns giving you the best of both worlds: the gentleness and elegance of permissive hypnosis; and the strength and reliability of direct authoritarian commands.

This blended style is what you will now learn as the Progressive Test Induction.

Why Both Styles Are Important

Although most modern hypnotherapy is conducted in a more Ericksonian style (while the client appears to remain awake), there are times when you want to lead your client into deeper levels of trance, particularly when you want:

- to install powerful post-hypnotic suggestions (e.g. stop smoking, weight management, healing)

- the client to forget the content of the suggestions (to prevent conscious interference)

- to access deep unconscious processes more easily.

In these cases, using authoritarian suggestions about sleep, combined with gentle permissiveness can create the perfect pathway.

How the Progressive Test Induction Works

The Progressive Test Induction follows a clear progression, incorporating tests at each stage to confirm the depth of the client's trance and build rapport with their unconscious mind. The induction is built around a series of tests that allow both you and your client to notice the natural deepening of trance. This includes:

- locked eyelids

- stiffened arms

- weak legs

- automatic movement

- sleep talking

- sleep walking

- visual hallucinations.

Each successful test acts as positive feedback, proving to the client that hypnosis is happening, and encouraging them to go even deeper.

And here's an important point: Even if a client doesn't succeed perfectly at one level, you simply move on because many clients will succeed more easily at deeper levels.

Hypnosis is not about passing or failing; it's about leading the client gradually inward.

Important Principles for Using the Progressive Test Induction

Here are some critical things to remember as you use this method.

1. Relax and Have Fun

This induction is meant to be playful, light-hearted and enjoyable. The more relaxed you are, the easier it will be for your client to relax and succeed. Remember, "anything that assumes trance produces trance".

2. Use Utilisation

If anything unexpected happens, such as a noise or a movement, use it. Utilisation means turning distractions into deepening opportunities. If the client does not produce the expected trance phenomena at one of the levels, utilise whatever the client does instead and move on to the next level.

3. Flow Between Styles

You'll begin with permissive language — "You might notice ..." — and gradually move into more direct suggestions — "Now your eyelids are locked tightly shut." This seamless blending makes the trance feel natural, not forced.

4. Focus on Deepening, Not Testing

Remember, these tests are NOT about passing or failing; they are about helping the client naturally experience deeper states of trance. If a test doesn't produce a full response, simply move forward smoothly.

5. Adjust for Each Client

Some clients may want to 'play' with the phenomena. Others may skip straight into very deep trance. Both are perfectly fine. Always tailor your pacing to the person in front of you. Repeat or expand on sentences as needed to assist the client into total relaxation.

6. Know When to Deliver Suggestions

Once your client has reached a suitably deep state, you can insert positive therapeutic/post hypnotic suggestions and produce amnesia of those suggestions. At this point, the Unconscious Mind is highly receptive.

7. Remove Suggestions Before Emerging

Before bringing the client out of trance, always remove any 'test' suggestions you installed. For example, remove suggestions like "your legs won't move" or "your arms are stiff" so the client returns to full, normal functioning afterward.

A Few Final Notes on Deep Trance

Some clients will naturally enter very deep states (even into a comatose-like state). Others will respond best at lighter or medium depths. Deep trance is not always necessary for effective hypnosis — what matters is communication with the Unconscious Mind.

If your client becomes very still or non-responsive at deep levels, you can gently request: "I'd like to ask your Unconscious Mind to send just enough energy to the parts of your body that need it for this process ... while keeping you comfortably deep inside."

The Progressive Test Induction Script

Please study and practice the Progressive Test Induction Script that follows. Feel free to repeat or expand sections as needed, based on your client's responses. The art of hypnosis lives in how flexibly you apply the structure.

Outline:

1. Close eyes — talk sleep

2. Eyelids locked closed

3. Stiff arms

4. Weak legs

5. Automatic movement

6. Talking in your sleep

7. Sleep walking

8. Visual hallucinations

9. Insert necessary suggestions here

10. Bring them out (remove suggestions)

Introduction:

"This induction is a fun test of your ability to reach the different levels of hypnosis and to actualise all the trance phenomena. It's set up with a number of tests, and the more tests you pass, the deeper you can go. So, enjoy it and let your Unconscious record everything so you don't have to pay total conscious attention to me as you go into a trance and you will be able to do it with your clients when you're ready to go ahead."

1. Close Eyes — Talk Sleep

"Now, if you would like to just go ahead and see if you can close your eyes. And I wonder if you can imagine, everybody can, imagining is something you can do, remember how much you imagined when you were little, or you can just remember a time when you were falling asleep (yawn), just falling sound asleep. Now, perhaps you can remember a time when you were soooo tired and relax(ed) ... all your muscles totally ... relax(ed) ... and just remember a time when you were falling asleep, going into a deep sleep. Deeper and deeper and deeper. Now, this is important, you can stay asleep as long as you want to stay asleep until I tell you and remember you will always hear the sound of my voice, however far or deep you go and you will always feel just fine and be just fine as a result of these suggestions. So, it's okay, just go ahead and fall sound, sound asleep. Deeper and deeper and deeper and deeper asleep. [*Continue deepening for 5 minutes.*] You may or may not remember to forget everything that happens, it's okay."

2. Eyelids Locked Closed

"Now, listen. Your eyelids, as deep as you are, you still know your eyes are closed and you may not have noticed that your eyelids feel so heavy that they are and they really ARE locked so tightly together that you may find it quite amusing to discover that your eyes are locked tight, tight, tight together. Your eyelids are locked tightly together and you can't open your eyes no matter how hard you try and REALLY try, the tighter they become. And you might care to try, so go ahead, I dare you to try and find with some amusement that you can't."

Relaxation: "Now, relax everything. Relax your eyelids. They are returning to normal and you are sound asleep. Sound, sound asleep and will sleep until I tell you. Then you will awaken quietly and easily, until then, just relax everything and sleep, sleep, sleep."

3. Stiff Arms

"Okay, it's time for our next test. So, just notice your right arm, right where it is [describe] becoming stiff and rigid, rigid and stiff. Stiff and rigid. And everyone knows how a piece of iron feels, so rigid and stiff, just like you ... can't bend your right arm. It's as if it were an iron bar, solid, rigid and stiff. It is impossible to bend your right arm, so stiff. I dare you to find with some amusement you can't."

Relaxation: "Now relax everything. Relax your arms. They are returning to normal and you are sound asleep. Sound, sound asleep and will sleep until I tell you. Then you will awaken quietly and easily, until then, just relax everything and sleep, sleep, sleep."

4. Weak Legs

"Now, even though you never thought of this before, now, notice it's as if your body is floating away, floating away, floating away. And you may discover with some delight that you cannot control your muscles in your legs, you are so relax(ed), now. And where were you born? Do you remember? Remember! Being a little newborn baby ... And now, like then, are stuck where you are and your legs won't work, too relax(ed). It is impossible for you to even try to stand up, too relaxed. And the harder you may try, the more relax(ed) your legs. You are just stuck there in the chair. You may try, and really try, I dare you."

Relaxation: "Now relax everything. Relax your legs. They are returning to normal and you are sound asleep. Sound, sound asleep and will sleep until I tell you. Then you will awaken quietly and easily, until then, just relax everything and sleep, sleep, sleep."

5. Automatic Movement

"Now listen carefully, more fun. It's time for us to discover just what your hands can do [*establish arm catalepsy.*] Now, let's start your hands rotating. Here they go [*start them rotating.*] Here they go, round and around. Faster and faster. Can your Unconscious ... keep them moving. They ARE rotating faster and faster, faster and faster. And you just might find with some delight you can't stop them. You can't stop, no matter how hard you try, the harder you try the faster they go around and around."

Relaxation: "Now relax everything. Relax your arms and hands. They are returning to normal and you are sound asleep. Sound, sound asleep and will sleep until I tell you. Then you will awaken quietly and easily, until then, just relax everything and sleep, sleep, sleep."

6. Talking in Your Sleep

"Now, I want you to dream and REALLY dream of talking in your sleep. Everyone knows of someone who talk(ed) in your sleep. So, sleep and have that dream. Now, I am going to ask you a few simple questions and you can just remain asleep in your dream and dream you answer me in your sleep talking in your sleep as you have seen people talk in your sleep. Soon I'm going to ask a question you will find it easy to answer. Okay, here it is:

- What is your name? Where do you live?

- Do you have any brothers or sisters?" [Avoid emotional questions.]

Relaxation: "Now relax everything. Relax your head, mouth and jaw. They are returning to normal and you are sound asleep. Sound, sound asleep and will sleep until I tell you. Then you will awaken quietly and easily, until then, just relax everything and sleep, sleep, sleep and continue to dream."

7. Sleep Walking

"In a moment, you will stand up. I will help you. You will remain asleep as you stand up, as if you were in a dream. You have seen sleepwalkers. Finding it easy (help subject) to stand up, go ahead, stand up. Walk. You are finding it easy to use your leg muscles as you remain deeply asleep. Standing up." [*Seat the client.*]

Relaxation: "Now relax everything. Relax your back and legs. They are returning to normal and you are sound asleep. Sound, sound asleep and will sleep until I tell you. Then you will awaken quietly and easily, until then, just relax everything and sleep, sleep, sleep."

8. Visual Hallucinations

"Now, listen carefully. In a moment, you're going to awaken from the neck up only. Your mind can remain asleep and your body can remain asleep, just your head with no recognition of your body can awaken from the neck up. When you're ready, just open your eyes. Open them now and remain deeply asleep. You are still dreaming and I want you to dream of this tennis ball. Open your eyes and look at the tennis ball in my hand. What colour is it?" [*Throw it up to see if subject follows the ball. Give ball to subject.*]

Relaxation: "Now relax everything. Relax your eyes and head. They are returning to normal and you are sound asleep. Sound, sound asleep and will sleep until I tell you. Then you will awaken quietly and easily, until then, just relax everything and sleep, sleep, sleep."

For demonstration purposes, you may choose to add Full Body Catalepsy into the Progressive Test Induction at this point.

Full Body Catalepsy is an advanced hypnotic phenomenon where the client's entire body becomes rigid and can even be supported horizontally between two chairs.

However, because Full Body Catalepsy requires extreme care, precise setup, and careful physical handling, it is more commonly taught during advanced hypnotherapy training rather than used in typical client sessions.

If you would like to safely learn and practice Full Body Catalepsy under expert supervision, this technique is taught during our Master Practitioner Certification Training.

Please remember: the safety, comfort, and wellbeing of your client must always come first.

9. Insert Additional Suggestions/Post Hypnotic Suggestions Here

Insert the necessary positive instructions and suggestions here. At this point, the suggestions should be direct.

NOTE: When working with post hypnotic suggestions, one of the most important elements for the successful actualisation of the suggestion is amnesia. This means that the client will not have recall of the suggestion when they emerge out of their trance. The client will experience an undeniable urge to actualise the behaviours embedded within the suggestion when the trigger moment arrives.

Amnesia for the suggestion can be created by using the "Remember to Forget" paradigm. Here's an example (you can create your own content to best fit your client):

"You went to a networking event and met lots of people. They gave you their business cards with their name on them. Do you remember the names of everyone you met? No, you forgot. It's okay to forget, remember to forget, it's easy, just forget, it's okay to forget, remember to forget ...

What did you have for dinner two weeks ago on a Tuesday? Do you remember? No, you forgot, that's good, it's okay to forget, too much information to be bothered with, remember to forget, it's okay to forget, it's natural, forget, forget, remember to forget ...

You have the phone numbers of many people. Can you remember them all? Of course not, you dial them and forget. It's okay to forget, it's natural, why bother to remember? It's okay to forget. You do it all the time, you can do it now, forget, forget, forget, remember to forget ..."

Continue if required.

Place the Post-Hypnotic Suggestion here

(Insert the necessary positive instructions and suggestions here. At this point, the suggestions should be direct.)

"Those phone numbers, you just won't remember, will you? No. You can forget, easily and effortlessly, it's good to forget. Remember to forget, it's okay to forget, remember to forget ...

Dinner two weeks ago on a Tuesday, why remember, it's not important, you can forget, it's easy to forget. It's okay to forget, remember to forget, right now ...

All those names on business cards, you have no call to remember them, it's okay to forget, forget, forget, it's okay to forget, forget now. You have no need for the memory, forget, it's okay to forget, remember to forget, forget now, that's right."

10. Bring Them Out

Remove any test or short-term suggestions here: "any and all suggestions about this trance and all related phenomena are hereby removed. All on-going suggestions are still in force." Count them out of trance. "In a moment, I am going to count backwards from 10 to 1, and I want you to awaken one tenth of the way with each number until you are fully awake. 10 ... 9 ... 8 ...", etc.

Key Points

The Progressive Test Induction:

- combines Ericksonian permissiveness with direct traditional suggestions

- leads the client naturally through deeper stages of trance

- builds belief and responsiveness through enjoyable "tests"

- teaches both the hypnotist and the client how powerful unconscious processes truly are.

Practise this method until it becomes second nature. The balance of structure and adaptability makes it an invaluable tool for any hypnotherapist. By mastering this induction, you'll be able to hypnotise almost anyone with elegance, confidence and ease.

Chapter 17:

Writing Hypnotic Suggestions that Create Real Change

One of the most powerful skills a hypnotherapist can develop is the ability to write clear, effective and emotionally resonant hypnotic suggestions. These suggestions become the 'change statements' your client hears during trance and often act as the blueprint for their transformation. In this chapter, you'll learn exactly how to craft suggestions that are tailored to your client's needs, are rooted in hypnotic principles and are delivered with maximum impact.

Why It Matters

Have you ever read a generic hypnosis script online and felt it lacked something? You're not alone. While some scripts may be helpful, others can be vague, poorly worded or even counterproductive. To become a confident and competent hypnotherapist, it's essential that you can write your own suggestions that are bespoke to the client, emotionally engaging, aligned with the client's goals and structured using powerful hypnotic patterns.

This chapter will walk you through that process.

The Difference Between Hypnotic Language Patterns and Hypnotic Suggestions

Before we begin, let's clear up a common confusion. Many students mix up Milton Model language patterns (which are used throughout a session to build trance, soften communication, and bypass resistance) with the actual hypnotic suggestions (the content inserted into the client's Unconscious for change). Milton Patterns are like the soil — they prepare the ground, soften resistance and create the right environment for growth. The hypnotic suggestion is the seed you plant in that soil. Good soil makes it easier for the seed to take root, but the seed itself is what grows into transformation.

The Five Golden Rules for Writing Hypnotic Suggestions (SPARK)

Use these **SPARK** rules as your checklist when writing any suggestion:

S – Specific

Vague suggestions are weak. Specific ones stick. Use words that create clear images, strong emotional resonance and a visceral sense of change.

For example: "You weigh between 65 and 69 kilos and love moving your body each day. You feel light, energised and vibrant." OR "You are comfortably within your ideal weight range and feel light, energised and vibrant."

Focus on what your client will see, hear and feel when the change has taken place. Use descriptive, emotionally rich language, like radiant, vibrant, glowing, relaxed, delightful, strong, clear, motivated, confident and joyful.

P – Positive

Your suggestion should always focus on what the client wants, not what they want to avoid. The Unconscious Mind does not process negatives effectively.

Instead of "You no longer feel nervous," use "You feel calm, confident, and centred."

Avoid words like can't, don't, never, not, try, tense, nervous, anxious and failure.

A – As If Now (Present Tense)

Speak your suggestion as though it is already happening. Avoid "will be" or "want to". Use phrases like:

"as you notice now ...", "you already experience ..." and "you enjoy the feeling of ..."

R – Realistic

Aim high but not impossibly high. Your suggestions should stretch the client just enough to excite and inspire them but remain believable to their Unconscious.

For example: "You naturally and easily choose foods that nourish your body. Every day you feel stronger and healthier."

Also, include the actions they will take, not just the outcomes.

K – Keep Repeating

Repetition builds conviction. Say the same message in different ways throughout the suggestion. This reinforces the idea while offering the Unconscious Mind multiple representations.

For example: "You enjoy healthy food. You naturally make nourishing choices. Eating well feels easy. You crave what supports your health."

Use at least three versions of the message.

Structure of a Hypnotic Suggestion

A well-formed suggestion is like a good sandwich:

- The first slice of bread is your setup (an induction and deepening script, Milton Model language, metaphors).

- The filling is your SPARK-based statement of change (the suggestion).

- The second slice of bread is your reinforcement and integration.

An example of the filling: "You now easily feel calm and composed when speaking in front of others. You enjoy sharing your ideas clearly and confidently. With each experience, your confidence grows, and you feel proud of your ability to stay relaxed, focused and effective. It feels natural now to stand tall and let your voice be heard."

Words to Avoid (and Use)

Avoid:

- negative words (no, not, can't, never, try)

- emotionally triggering words (anxious, fail, nervous, struggle)

Use:

- emotionally positive words (radiant, delighted, calm, confident, strong, vibrant)

- sensory-based words (see, feel, notice, sense, hear)

- empowering language (naturally, easily, now, fully, freely)

Common Mistakes to Avoid

- Writing about what the client doesn't want

- Overcomplicating the suggestion with too many ideas

- Being too general or vague

- Forgetting to connect the change with emotion and sensory experience

Practice Exercise: Write Your Own Suggestion

Now it's your turn. Use this process to write a suggestion for yourself. Choose a goal or outcome that you'd like to achieve (e.g. weight loss, confidence, better sleep, motivation, letting go of a habit, etc.).

Follow the 5 SPARK rules: **Specific, Positive, As If Now, Realistic, Keep Repeating**

For example: "You are calm and confident every time you prepare to speak. Your breathing is steady and relaxed. You feel focused and strong. You enjoy the feeling of clarity in your voice. Speaking in front of others comes easily and naturally to you now."

Now write your own.

Once you've written it, read it out loud. Notice how it makes you feel. Ask yourself:

- does it feel good?

- does it follow SPARK?

- would it excite your client if they heard it?

Refine it as you go.

And remember — great suggestions create great results.

Welcome to the part of hypnosis where the words you choose really do become the results your clients experience.

Chapter 18:

The Art of Utilisation

What is Utilisation and Why is it Important?

Utilisation is one of the most effective and versatile tools you can use as a hypnotherapist. First developed and refined by Milton Erickson, utilisation is the art of using everything that happens — within the client or the environment — to deepen trance and make your suggestions even more powerful.

In traditional hypnosis, earlier practitioners would often take a directive approach, saying things like, "Uncross your legs. Take a deep breath. Close your eyes." While this style can work, it can also create resistance in clients who do not respond well to authoritarian methods. Erickson discovered that instead of fighting against what naturally happens, a hypnotherapist can guide the client by utilising their responses, behaviours and surroundings to deepen trance naturally.

Why Utilisation Works

The beauty of utilisation lies in its flexibility. Instead of ignoring or avoiding distractions, unexpected events or the client's own unique responses, utilisation turns those elements into tools for creating deeper rapport and trance. Whether the client blinks, shifts position, breathes a little more deeply or notices a sound in the room, these moments can be woven into the trance experience.

The key to mastering utilisation is to observe the client closely and respond to what you notice. When you acknowledge something the client is doing —

even unconsciously — it builds rapport and signals to the Unconscious Mind that you are in tune with their experience.

Examples of Utilisation

Imagine you are working with a client, and they blink naturally. You could say: *"That's right. As you blink, you might start to notice how easy it is to let your eyes feel heavier now."*

Or, if a clock chimes or a noise occurs in the room, you might say: *"That sound can remind you of how quickly you can go even deeper ... now."*

These statements validate the client's experience and subtly incorporate the environment into the session, reinforcing the hypnotic state.

Erickson's Mastery of Utilisation

Milton Erickson was a master at utilisation. He would notice even the smallest changes in his clients — like a slight shift in breathing, a tiny movement of the hand or a fixed gaze — and use those observations to deepen trance.

He might say: *"I don't know if you've noticed this yet, but your breathing has already started to slow ... and that might mean you're relaxing more comfortably than you expected."*

By pointing out what is already happening, Erickson gave the client's Unconscious Mind the suggestion that the process was unfolding perfectly. This builds confidence in both the hypnotherapist and the experience of trance itself.

How to Use Utilisation in Practice

Here are key strategies for using utilisation effectively in your sessions:

1. Pay Attention to the Client

- Observe subtle changes in breathing, posture, eye movements or facial expressions.

- Notice any natural or automatic actions, such as a swallow, blink or slight relaxation of the muscles.

2. Utilise the Environment

- If there's background noise, integrate it into the session: *"That sound outside can remind you to go deeper into your own comfort."*

- If there is light filtering through a window, use it: *"The light gently filtering in can help you feel calm and present."*

3. Use Simple Acknowledgments

A simple, *"That's right,"* after noticing something the client does, reinforces their Unconscious response and builds rapport. For example: *"That's right … as you take another breath, you can feel even more relaxed."*

4. Turn Challenges into Opportunities

- If a client fidgets or appears distracted, you might say: *"As you shift in your chair, you can settle even more comfortably now."*

- If they seem unsure about the process, you can utilise that: *"It's okay to wonder whether this is working … because wondering often leads to even deeper relaxation."*

Convincers: Proving the Reality of Trance

Sometimes clients are surprised that trance feels so natural. They may question whether they were actually in trance at all. This is where convincers come into play. A convincer is an experience or demonstration that shows the client their Unconscious Mind has responded to your suggestions.

For example:

- **Arm Catalepsy**: ask the client to raise their arm and then suggest that it becomes stiff and rigid. After the arm remains in position, you can ask them to open their eyes and notice it. This creates a powerful realisation: *"You're doing that, and your Unconscious Mind is responding perfectly."*

- **Blink Suggestion:** You might say, *"In a moment, you'll blink—and as you do, you can relax even more."* When the client blinks, you follow up with, *"That's right,"* reinforcing that they are responding to your suggestions.

These small demonstrations confirm to the client that trance is real and that their Unconscious Mind is engaged in the process.

Practical Exercise: Mastering Utilisation

Here's a simple exercise you can practise with a partner to build your skills in utilisation.

1. Set Up: one person is the hypnotherapist, and the other is the client. The hypnotherapist sits at a comfortable angle, ideally between 90 to 135 degrees, to the client.

Why this angle matters:

Sitting at a 90–135 degree angle is ideal for hypnosis and deep trance work. It allows the client to feel unobserved and safe, encouraging them to turn their focus inward rather than feeling watched. This non-confrontational positioning also builds unconscious rapport by creating a gentle, side-by-side presence.

By contrast, a 45–90 degree angle is slightly more front-facing and conversational. It's often useful during coaching or NLP sessions, especially when clients are talking through ideas or engaging the Conscious Mind.

In short:

- 90–135° is best for trance, regression, or inner work.

- 45–90° is useful for pre-talk, debrief, or coaching-style interactions.

You can observe your client's response to each angle and adapt intuitively. The goal is always comfort, trust and flow.

2. Observe and Utilise: the hypnotherapist observes any natural actions or signs of relaxation the client exhibits — a blink, a change in breathing, a shift in posture.

Each time something happens, the hypnotherapist says, "That's right," and follows up with a suggestion like *"As you blink, you might notice yourself going even deeper."*

3. Switch Roles: after five minutes, reverse roles so that both participants get to experience utilisation as both the hypnotherapist and the client.

Why Utilisation is Essential

Utilisation is not just a technique, it's a mindset. It invites you to trust that everything in the session has potential value, and it teaches you to work with the client's natural responses rather than against them. Every movement, every behaviour, every word and even every distraction is an opportunity to deepen trance and enhance the therapeutic process.

When you master utilisation, you:

- build deeper rapport with your clients

- create a sense of flow and naturalness in your sessions

- reinforce the client's belief in their ability to go into trance and accept suggestions.

Moving Forward

In hypnotherapy, everything that happens has value — if you know how to utilise it. By observing closely, responding naturally and weaving suggestions into the client's experience, you will become a confident and resourceful hypnotherapist. As you continue your training, you will refine your utilisation skills further, integrating them seamlessly with other techniques to achieve profound results for your clients.

Remember: Utilise, utilise, utilise. When you do, every moment becomes an opportunity for transformation.

Chapter 19:

The Power of Milton Model Patterns

Why Language Matters in Hypnotherapy

A thorough understanding of both hypnosis and Neuro-Linguistic Programming (NLP) is essential for becoming a skilled and versatile hypnotherapist. One of the most powerful tools you can develop as a hypnotherapist is the ability to use language intentionally and effectively. Milton H. Erickson, a legendary figure in hypnosis, revolutionised how language could create deep rapport with the Unconscious Mind through his Milton Model Language Patterns.

Earlier hypnotists used direct, authoritarian instructions like, *"Uncross your legs. Put your hands on your thighs. Take a deep breath and close your eyes"*. Erickson, however, developed a permissive and conversational style; an approach that allowed clients to enter trance effortlessly, often without realising they were being guided.

For those new to hypnotherapy, understanding these patterns can feel overwhelming at first. But rest assured that you'll be guided step by step. You will also see how these hypnotic patterns connect deeply with NLP, enabling you to use language to influence, heal and empower. In our NLP Practitioner and NLP Master Practitioner programs, you will explore these tools further. By the time you reach our NLP Trainers Training, you will be able to use them with precision and volition, effortlessly integrating them into your communication.

How Milton Erickson Transformed Hypnosis

Milton Erickson understood that the Unconscious Mind responds to ambiguity. When language becomes intentionally vague or layered, the Unconscious begins to search for meaning, creating a natural opening for trance. Erickson often started with a simple, conversational question like: "I wonder, as you sit there and listen to my voice, if you can begin to feel yourself becoming more comfortable ... now."

Notice how this statement feels more like a suggestion than a command. Instead of demanding a specific response, it gently invites the listener to relax. This conversational tone bypasses resistance and allows the Unconscious Mind to follow along without objection.

Key Milton Model Patterns and Simple Examples

Here is an introduction to the Milton Model patterns with examples that are easy to understand for beginners.

1. Mind Read

Claiming to know someone's thoughts or feelings.

- *"I know you're curious about how quickly you can relax."*

- Why it works: this draws the listener's attention inward, encouraging self-reflection.

2. Cause and Effect

Implying that one thing causes another.

- *"As you take a deep breath, you'll find your body beginning to relax."*

- Why it works: it links a simple action (breathing) to a desired outcome (relaxation).

3. Presupposition

An assumption embedded in a sentence.

- *"You can start to notice how calm you feel as you listen to my voice."*

- Why it works: the sentence assumes the person will feel calm, leading them toward that state.

4. Tag Question

A question added at the end of a sentence to invite agreement.

- *"It feels good to relax, doesn't it?"*

- Why it works: it encourages the listener to agree unconsciously.

5. Pacing Current Experience

Describing what someone is experiencing right now.

- *"You're sitting there, hearing my words, breathing in and out."*

- Why it works: it builds rapport by aligning with the listener's current reality.

6. Double Bind

Offering two choices that lead to the same outcome.

- *"You can relax now, or you can relax in a few moments—it's entirely up to you."*

- Why it works: both choices support the goal (relaxation), giving the listener a sense of control.

7. Ambiguity

Using language with multiple interpretations to engage the Unconscious Mind.

- *"I don't know if you'll relax first in your shoulders... or in your breathing."*

- Why it works: It keeps the listener's mind searching for meaning, encouraging trance.

Putting the Patterns Together

Here's an example of how you might combine Milton Model patterns into a short induction.

"I know you've been wondering about how good it might feel to truly relax, haven't you? And as you listen to the sound of my voice, you might start to notice your breathing slowing down ... and the muscles in your shoulders beginning to let go. You can take your time ... or just go even deeper now ... because that sense of comfort can spread as easily as it needs to."

You can find all the key components in this example.

- Mind Read: *"I know you've been wondering..."*

- Tag Question: *"...haven't you?"*

- Pacing: *"...as you listen to the sound of my voice..."*

- Cause and Effect (Pacing statement plus): *"...you might start to notice your breathing slowing down."*

- Double Bind: *"You can take your time... or just go even deeper now."*

Why Milton Model Patterns Matter for Beginners

For those new to hypnotherapy, the Milton Model provides a powerful way to create connection and trust with your clients' Unconscious Minds. Unlike direct, authoritarian approaches, Ericksonian language patterns feel natural, gentle and permissive. They allow clients to experience trance in a way that feels safe, comfortable and empowering.

In most trainings, these patterns are taught progressively. In NLP Practitioner Training, you will learn how to recognise and begin using the full set of Milton Model Language Patterns. In the NLP Master Practitioner Training, you will refine your ability to layer language patterns for deeper therapeutic results. By the time you complete NLP Trainers Training, you will be able to use these tools with volition — adapting them effortlessly to meet any situation or client need.

Practice: Experience the Patterns Yourself

To begin exploring the Milton Model, try this simple exercise:

1. Pick one or two patterns, such as Mind Read and Pacing Current Experience.

2. Write a few sentences you might say to someone to help them relax, using these patterns.

3. Practise saying these sentences aloud in a calm, soothing tone.

For example:

- *"I know you might already be feeling more comfortable, just sitting there and reading these words.*

- *"You're breathing naturally, and as you read this sentence, you might start to notice how relaxed your hands feel."*

As you practise, notice how these patterns feel to you. The more familiar you become with the Milton Model, the easier it will be to use these tools naturally and effectively.

The 19 Milton Model Patterns

The Milton Model comprises 19 powerful language patterns that enable hypnotherapists to create deep rapport and guide clients into transformative states. These patterns include tools like Mind Reads, Pacing Statements, Presuppositions, Tag Questions, Ambiguities, and many more.

You will learn all 19 patterns in detail during your NLP Practitioner and Master Practitioner Trainings, where you will master their application to both hypnosis and everyday communication. By the time you reach NLP Trainers Training, you will be using these patterns fluently, understanding how to layer them for maximum effectiveness. For now, let's explore two additional tools: Leading Statements and Embedded Commands.

Leading Statements and Embedded Commands

A leading statement is a suggestion that gently guides a person toward a desired state or action. When combined with pacing statements —

descriptions of the client's current undeniable reality — leading statements can bypass resistance and create a pathway for change.

An embedded command is a directive subtly hidden within a larger sentence. These commands are often marked by a slight pause or change in tonality, which signals the Unconscious Mind to pay attention. Erickson often used embedded commands to encourage clients to act on suggestions without consciously resisting.

Here's how these patterns work together:

1. Start with 3 pacing statements to build rapport and describe the client's current experience.

2. Follow with a leading statement or embedded command to guide the client toward the desired outcome.

Example of Pacing and Leading with Embedded Commands

Let's look at a simple example to help you understand: "You are sitting here, listening to my voice ... feeling your body supported by the chair ... breathing in and out naturally ... and you might begin to feel more relaxed ... now."

- Pacing Statements: *"You are sitting here, listening to my voice ... feeling your body supported by the chair ... breathing in and out naturally."* These statements describe the client's undeniable reality, building trust and rapport.

- Leading Statement/Embedded Command: *"... and you might begin to feel more relaxed ... now."* The embedded command *"feel more relaxed now"* is subtle and inviting, directing the client's Unconscious Mind toward relaxation.

Another Example

For a client experiencing stress, you might say:

"You've been working hard all week ... noticing how much you've been doing ... and taking this time now to sit back and relax ... allows you to let go ... completely."

- Pacing Statements: *"You've been working hard all week ... noticing how much you've been doing ... and taking this time now to sit back and relax."*

- Embedded Command: *"... allows you to let go ... completely."*

Here, the pacing statements align with the client's reality, while the embedded command *"let go completely"* encourages relaxation at an Unconscious level.

For beginners, combining pacing statements with leading statements and embedded commands is an easy, yet highly effective, way to guide clients into trance. By starting with the client's current experience, you build trust and reduce resistance. Then, you subtly guide them toward relaxation, healing or positive change.

As you practise these tools, you will begin to see how small shifts in language can create profound changes. The Milton Model provides a flexible, conversational approach to hypnosis that feels natural for both the client and the hypnotherapist.

Practice Exercise

To begin practising, try this:

1. Pick a situation, such as guiding someone to relax.

2. Write three pacing statements that describe what the person is experiencing.

- For example: "You are sitting comfortably ... breathing gently ... noticing the sounds around you."

3. Follow with a leading statement or embedded command.

- For example: "... and you can begin to feel more calm and centered."

4. Practise saying it aloud with a soft, steady tone, emphasising the embedded command.

Moving Forward

The Milton Model Language Patterns are the key to mastering conversational hypnosis and creating deep, meaningful change. In the trainings to come, we will delve even deeper into these patterns, teaching you how to combine them seamlessly to become a confident, effective hypnotherapist.

Remember: language is powerful and when used with intention, it can transform lives.

Chapter 20:

Ericksonian Interventions

The purpose of our first two Ericksonian inductions (Chapter 15) was to provide practice for you, the hypnotherapist, in inducing trance and guiding your client into learning how to enter a trance state. In this chapter, we will take your skills further by focusing on Ericksonian interventions that facilitate real and lasting change for your client.

These interventions use a combination of Milton Erickson's indirect suggestions, The Release System™, and specific NLP techniques, creating a powerful synergy to address both generalised and specific issues. This integrated approach equips you to confidently adapt your sessions to your client's unique needs.

The General Hypnosis Paradigm

Milton Erickson believed that every client has the resources they need to resolve their problems within their Unconscious Mind. The role of the hypnotherapist is to help the client access those resources, overcome obstacles and facilitate healing or transformation.

The General Hypnosis Paradigm gives you a clear structure for conducting a successful hypnotherapy session. It consists of five key stages:

1. Preparation

2. Induction

3. Utilisation

4. Change Work

5. Bringing the Client Out of Trance

This process is flexible and can be tailored to fit almost any client and problem.

1. Preparation

- Define the desired outcome: Ask the client what they want to change or achieve. Ensure their goals are positive, clear and measurable.

- Obtain personal history: Use the personal history questions from Chapter 9 to uncover the presenting problem and any patterns or underlying causes.

- Pre-talk and suggestibility tests: Eliminate misconceptions about hypnosis and conduct suggestibility tests to build the client's confidence in their ability to enter trance.

2. Induction

Choose an induction that suits the client. Ericksonian methods, such as the Arm Levitation Induction from Chapter 15, are excellent because they are permissive, indirect and flexible.

3. Utilisation

Utilise everything the client does or says during trance to deepen their experience. Pay attention to physiological signs (e.g. relaxed breathing, eye fluttering) to gauge the depth of trance. Respond with *"That's right"* to validate and encourage trance behaviours.

4. Change Work: 6 Steps for Ericksonian Intervention

This is where the actual transformation happens. Once the client is in a trance, follow these steps to elicit their Unconscious Mind's cooperation and facilitate healing or change.

- Step 1: Does your Unconscious Mind know what to do to solve the problem?

Ask: *"Does your Unconscious Mind know what to do to solve this problem?"*

If the client answers *"yes"*, acknowledge it as a sign that rapport has been established with their Unconscious Mind.

If the answer is *"no"*, you can say: *"Can your Unconscious Mind get in touch with the blueprint of perfect health and healing that exists in your Higher Self and transfer it to your body?"*

- Step 2: Is it possible for your Unconscious Mind to heal the condition?

Ask: *"Is it possible for your Unconscious Mind to heal this now?"*

If the client says "no", remind their Unconscious Mind of its purpose: *"Your Unconscious Mind has always taken care of you — breathing, healing cuts, regulating your heart. It can heal this, too, can't it?"*

- Step 3: Is it alright to heal this now or to organise the steps now for healing?

Ask: *"Is it alright for your Unconscious Mind to heal this now or organise the steps to heal it?"*

If there is resistance, gently reframe it: *"Sometimes the Unconscious Mind holds onto things out of habit, but its ultimate purpose is to protect you. Wouldn't it feel wonderful to let this go now?"*

- Step 4: Are there any other problems your Unconscious Mind would like to work on?

Ask: *"Are there any other problems your Unconscious Mind would like to work on today?"*

This step allows the client's Unconscious to address additional concerns. If the answer is 'yes', repeat steps 1 to 4, asking the questions to 'all the problems'.

- Step 5: Unconscious Mind, go ahead and heal (client's name).

Give permission directly to the Unconscious Mind: *"Unconscious Mind, go ahead and heal [client's name] now, in the perfect way and at the perfect time."*

- Step 6: How quickly will your Unconscious Mind start the healing? How quickly will it finish?

Ask: *"How quickly will your Unconscious Mind start the healing? How quickly will it finish?"*

Provide positive options: *"Sometimes the Unconscious likes to start right away, and sometimes it begins in a few hours. Which would you prefer?"*

5. Bringing the Client Out of Trance

Use a gentle count-out: *"In a moment, I'm going to count backwards from 10 to 1. With each number, you'll become more alert, more awake, and fully aware. 10 … 9 … 8 … starting to feel refreshed … 7 … 6 … 5 … taking a nice, deep breath … 4 … 3 … becoming aware of the room … 2 … and 1. Wide awake, feeling wonderful!"*

Case Study: Resolving a Fear of Public Speaking

Client Background: Sarah, a 35-year-old professional, came to hypnotherapy with a fear of public speaking that impacted her career. She had no specific traumatic event but described feeling nervous, breathless and blank whenever she spoke in front of groups.

Steps Taken in the Session

1. Preparation

- Sarah explained her desired outcome: *"I want to feel calm, confident and clear when speaking to an audience."*

- A pre-talk addressed myths about hypnosis, and suggestibility tests (e.g. Finger Vice) reassured Sarah she could enter trance.

2. Induction

- Used the Arm Levitation Induction, Sarah's breathing deepened and her hand began lifting automatically, indicating light trance.

3. Utilisation

- Observed her relaxed breathing and slight eye fluttering: *"That's right ... noticing how relaxed you feel as your body settles deeper into comfort."*

4. Change Work

- Step 1: *"Does your Unconscious Mind know what to do to help you feel calm when speaking?"* → Yes.

- Step 2: *"Is it possible for your Unconscious to let you feel confident and relaxed?"* → Yes.

- Step 3: *"Is it all right for you to make this change now?"* → *Sarah nodded.*

- Step 4: (We skipped step 4 in this instance.)

- Step 5: *"Unconscious Mind, go ahead and allow Sarah to feel calm, clear, and confident every time she speaks in public."*

- Step 6: *"How quickly will your Unconscious Mind start this change?"* → *"Now."*

5. Suggestions

- While in trance: "You'll feel a sense of calm spreading through your body every time you stand up to speak. Your breathing will slow, your voice will flow naturally and you'll feel excited to share your ideas."

6. Count Out

- Sarah emerged from trance feeling refreshed and positive.

Result: At a follow-up session, Sarah reported successfully giving a presentation at work: *"I felt calm, confident and even enjoyed it!"*

This case study illustrates how the General Hypnosis Paradigm and Ericksonian techniques can produce tangible, life-changing results. By learning to trust this process, you will develop the flexibility and confidence to assist clients with a wide range of challenges.

Key Notes

STEP 1: Does your Unconscious Mind know what to do to solve the problem?

The first step begins by inviting the client's Unconscious Mind to step into its natural role as a problem solver. This question bypasses the Conscious Mind, allowing the deeper resources of the Unconscious to begin working on the desired outcome.

Why It's Important

Many clients consciously feel stuck because they believe they don't know how to resolve their issue. By asking this question, you remind the client that their Unconscious Mind already holds the answers and solutions. This builds trust in the process and empowers the client.

How to Ask It

- "Does your Unconscious Mind know what to do to solve this problem?"

- Follow up with soft reinforcement: *"That's right ... your Unconscious Mind is so powerful, it has already stored everything you need to know to resolve this now."*

What to Do if the Answer is 'Yes'

If the client answers *"yes"*, affirm their response: *"That's perfect. Your Unconscious knows exactly what to do. And we can trust it to begin that process now, in its own perfect way."*

What to Do if the Answer is 'No'

If the client says *"no"*, or doesn't respond, reassure them that the answer is within their deeper mind:

1. Ask about the Higher Self: *"Can your Unconscious Mind connect now to the blueprint of perfect health and wisdom in your Higher Self... and allow that wisdom to help?"* This metaphor helps the client imagine a resourceful version of themselves with solutions already in place.

2. Invite Curiosity: *"That's okay. Sometimes the answers come when you least expect them, and you may find your Unconscious bringing forward just what you need as we continue."*

Practical Example

If a client wants to overcome procrastination but says their Unconscious doesn't know what to do:

- Say: *"That's okay. Your Unconscious Mind has so much experience helping you solve other challenges, hasn't it? Maybe it just needs to reconnect with the part of you that knows what it feels like to take action."*

- Pause to allow the Unconscious to process.

- Then gently reinforce: *"And as that connection happens now, you can begin to notice how ready you are for this change."*

STEP 2: Is it possible for your Unconscious Mind to heal the condition?

Here, you help the client's Unconscious Mind recognise that change is possible. This step is about reinforcing belief and opening a door to healing or transformation.

Why It's Important

Clients often hold limiting beliefs about their ability to change. By asking this question, you gently dissolve resistance and reframe the situation into one of possibility.

How to Ask It

- *"Is it possible for your Unconscious Mind to heal this condition or resolve this problem?"*

- Add a sense of certainty: *"Because when you really think about it, anything is possible when you let your Unconscious do what it does best."*

If the Answer is 'Yes'

Celebrate and encourage this belief: *"That's right. Your Unconscious Mind knows it's possible... and that's the first step toward making it happen."*

If the Answer is 'No' or Unclear

Gently redirect to possibility.

1. Use metaphor: *"Your body heals a cut all by itself ... and perhaps your Unconscious can begin healing this too, step by step."*

2. Ask about the Higher Self: *"Can your Unconscious Mind connect now to the blueprint of perfect health and wisdom in your Higher Self... and allow that wisdom to help?"* This metaphor helps the client imagine a resourceful version of themselves with solutions already in place.

3. Engage the imagination: *"If it were possible ... what would that look like or sound like or feel like?"*

Practical Example

For a client struggling with chronic stress:

- You: "Is it possible for your Unconscious Mind to begin releasing those feelings of stress now?"

- Client: "I'm not sure."

- You: "That's okay. Your body already knows how to relax, doesn't it? Just like when you drift into a peaceful sleep... your Unconscious can begin to release that tension now."

STEP 3: Is it alright to heal this now or to organise the steps now for healing?

This step gives the Unconscious Mind permission to move forward. Sometimes, clients unconsciously resist change due to emotional or ecological concerns, and this step gently addresses those blocks.

Why It's Important

For change to be lasting, the Unconscious Mind must accept that it is 'alright' to let go of the problem. This step aligns the client's desires with the deeper mind's sense of timing and purpose.

How to Ask It

- *"Is it alright to heal this now, or to organise the steps for healing?"*

- Add reassurance: *"Your Unconscious Mind knows the perfect time and way to let this happen, doesn't it?"*

What to Do if the Answer is 'No'

If the Unconscious says it's not ready, explore why:

1. Address positive purpose/intention: *"Sometimes a problem serves a purpose or intention we're not aware of. Would it be okay to release this problem and find a new, healthier way to fulfill that purpose?"*

2. Reframe timing: *"If not now, that's fine. Can your Unconscious begin preparing for the change, so it happens when it's ready?"*

Practical Example

If a client feels anxious about healing past trauma:

- You: "Is it all right for your Unconscious to start letting go of those old feelings now?"

- Client: "I'm not sure."

- You: "That's perfectly fine. Maybe it can begin organising the steps to let go, one small bit at a time, in a way that feels safe and gentle."

STEP 4: Are there any other problems your Unconscious Mind would like to work on?

This step is often overlooked, but it's a valuable opportunity for the Unconscious Mind to bring forward any other issues that may be related to the presenting problem. Often, a client comes to a session focused on a symptom rather than the root cause. By creating space for the Unconscious Mind to share additional concerns, you allow deeper healing to take place.

How to Know What Else There is to Work On

1. Listen to the client's language and clues

During the personal history or the pre-talk, pay close attention to subtle cues in the client's language, tone, and descriptions.

For example, a client working on stress relief might say, "I'm just so exhausted all the time, I can't focus. This hints that sleep quality and concentration might also need attention.

You can follow up with, *"I wonder if your Unconscious Mind is ready to address those feelings of exhaustion too."*

2. Trust the Unconscious Mind

The Unconscious Mind knows the full picture. You don't need to identify every issue consciously. Simply ask: *"Is there anything else your Unconscious Mind feels ready to work on today?"*

The Unconscious may respond with a feeling, an image or a simple sense of 'yes'

You can follow up with: *"What else would your Unconscious Mind like us to focus on?"*

If the client's Unconscious Mind isn't clear, trust that it will reveal itself as the work progresses.

3. Watch for hypnotic signals

Even in deep trance, subtle physical movements can signal that the Unconscious Mind is addressing something significant. These may include:

- a slight change in breathing

- movement of a hand or fingers (ideomotor responses)

- shifts in facial expressions.

If you notice these signals, you can say: *"It seems like there's something more your Unconscious is ready to bring forward … and you can allow that to happen now."*

4. Encourage collaboration

Frame this step as a cooperative effort with the Unconscious. This invites trust and openness.

For example: *"Your Unconscious has been so wonderful in helping you today. And perhaps it knows there's something else that, when released, will allow you to feel even better, even lighter."*

Practical Example

Let's say you're working with Sarah, a client who you're helping to overcome public speaking anxiety. Here's how Step 4 might unfold:

- You: "Is there anything else your Unconscious Mind wants to work on today?"

- Sarah (in trance): "I just feel this tension in my stomach … like there's something else."

- You: "That's right. You can trust that your Unconscious Mind knows exactly what this feeling is about … and that we can begin to work on that now, safely and comfortably."

As the tension is addressed, you may discover that the stomach feeling relates to fear of judgement rooted in earlier experiences. By allowing space for the Unconscious to reveal this, you're not only helping Sarah with her presenting issue (public speaking) but also releasing a deeper emotional block.

What to Do if Nothing Comes Up

Sometimes the Unconscious Mind may indicate that there's nothing else to work on. That's okay! Respect this response and reinforce it positively: *"That's perfect. Your Unconscious knows exactly what to work on and when, and you've done such wonderful work today."*

Why This Step Matters

By asking the Unconscious if there's anything else to address, you:

- prevent future 'symptom substitution', where a new problem arises after the initial one is resolved

- build deeper trust and communication with the client's Unconscious Mind

- ensure your client receives comprehensive and lasting results.

This step demonstrates that you're committed to supporting the client's overall well-being, not just the initial reason they walked into your office. It reflects an integrated approach to hypnotherapy: listening deeply, trusting the Unconscious and guiding clients to profound, transformative change.

STEP 5: Unconscious Mind, go ahead and heal (client's name)

This is the activation step, where you invite the client's Unconscious to take action. You are giving it permission and encouragement to follow through.

Why It's Important

It creates a clear directive for the Unconscious Mind to begin healing or making the desired change.

How to Ask It

You can say: *"Unconscious Mind, go ahead and begin healing (client's name) now."*

Remember to add supportive suggestions like: *"And as this happens, you can feel calm, peaceful and completely aligned."*

STEP 6: How quickly will the Unconscious Mind start the healing? How quickly will it finish?

This step is where we invite the Unconscious Mind to take intentional action by asking it to provide a clear timeframe for the healing or change process. While the Unconscious Mind is powerful, it operates on the path of least resistance — meaning it will always choose the simplest and most efficient route to achieve a result. This step ensures the Unconscious works deliberately and within a specific timeframe, allowing both you and the client to measure progress and success.

Why It's Important

The Unconscious Mind works well with clear parameters. By suggesting a timeline, you help clients feel a sense of progress and immediacy.

How to Ask It

Say: *"How quickly will your Unconscious Mind begin healing?"*

Then follow up with: *"Will it finish today, or in the perfect amount of time?"*

If the Client Seems Hesitant

Reassure them: *"Your Unconscious can begin as soon as it's ready. And when it's finished, you'll notice just how good it feels to have resolved this."*

Practical Example

For a client working on breaking a smoking habit:

- You: "How quickly will your Unconscious Mind begin to let go of that old habit now?"

- Client: "Right away."

- You: "That's perfect. And how soon will it be complete? Maybe today ... or by the time you wake up tomorrow."

Why Pinning Down Timeframes is Crucial

The body and mind function with natural rhythms and processes that are already happening at an unconscious level. By directing the Unconscious Mind to operate within a specified time, we align it with those natural processes, speeding up healing and change while ensuring the client can consciously observe results.

Understanding the natural regeneration of the body empowers hypnotherapists to communicate precise yet realistic expectations. This builds confidence in the process and helps the client trust that change is happening.

How the Body Regenerates Itself

Understanding the body's natural healing and renewal cycles is helpful when framing realistic timelines for the Unconscious Mind.

Modern biology shows that the human body is not a static structure but a dynamic system in continuous renewal. Many tissues and cells throughout the body regularly repair, regenerate and replace themselves as part of normal biological functioning.

By recognising these natural rhythms of renewal, the Unconscious Mind can organise and support healing processes in alignment with the body's inherent capacity for restoration.

The following examples illustrate some of the body's remarkable regenerative processes. They are used to help the Unconscious Mind organise healing responses and are not intended as medical diagnosis or treatment.

1. Skin regeneration: skin cells undergo a renewal process approximately every 28 days.

"Your Unconscious Mind can initiate this process now, recognising that in about a month, your skin can be entirely renewed, leading to a healthier and more vibrant appearance."

2. Liver renewal: the liver possesses a significant regenerative capacity, capable of replacing damaged cells over time.

"Your Unconscious Mind understands how to commence this healing, supporting the liver's natural repair and renewal processes and allowing the liver to function in a healthier and more balanced way."

3. Stomach lining: the stomach lining is known to renew itself every few days.

"In just a few days, your Unconscious Mind can completely restore and renew the stomach lining, promoting comfort and healthy digestive function."

4. Blood cells: red blood cells have a lifespan of about 120 days, with the body continually producing new ones.

"Your body is already in the process of renewing your blood cells daily, and your Unconscious Mind can ensure they carry vitality and health throughout your entire system."

5. Bone and cartilage: bone tissue undergoes continuous remodelling, with complete regeneration occurring over months to years, depending on various factors.

"Your Unconscious Mind can begin this healing process now, aligning with your body's natural rhythm to facilitate effective and harmonious recovery."

These natural cycles of renewal demonstrate that the human body is constantly repairing, replacing and reorganising itself. When the Unconscious Mind aligns with these biological processes, it can support the body's innate capacity for healing and restoration.

How to Pin the Unconscious Mind Down to Timeframes

The Unconscious Mind, while powerful, is often ambiguous unless directed with clear, specific suggestions. This is because it operates without linear time — it understands experiences, sensations and patterns, not the conscious sense of 'a week' or 'a month'. Therefore, your role is to introduce a timeframe that feels both reasonable and achievable for the client's healing journey.

Framing Timeframes Effectively

1. Start with immediate action: begin by suggesting the healing process starts now. This creates momentum and eliminates procrastination.

"Unconscious Mind, how quickly can you begin this healing? Perhaps it's starting now, in this very moment, or maybe as soon as the next breath you take."

2. Introduce specific timeframes: use physiological facts or familiar cycles to guide the Unconscious.

"The body already knows how to heal, and since a stomach lining renews itself in approx five days, your Unconscious Mind can start healing that discomfort today and finish within the next few days."

3. Create flexibility and safety: give the Unconscious Mind a choice to ease resistance while keeping it on track.

"How quickly will you finish? Perhaps it's as soon as tomorrow, or maybe over the next few days — whatever is healthiest and most effective for you."

4. Tie results to a positive outcome: reinforce the benefits of achieving the change within the given timeframe.

"By this time next week, you may already feel lighter, healthier and more energised as the healing completes itself beautifully and naturally."

Example of a Healing Dialogue

Use the following steps for a client working on stress-related digestion issues.

1. Immediate action

"Unconscious Mind, you can start the healing process now, as soon as this next breath, knowing the body naturally renews itself in ways that are perfectly aligned with health."

2. Introduce timeframe

"Since the stomach lining renews itself in as little as five days, the Unconscious Mind can complete this process in five days or even sooner, bringing calm, balance, and comfort."

3. Reinforce benefits

"You might already begin to notice how much better you feel tomorrow or the next day, and by the end of the week, that sensation of comfort and relaxation can be your new normal."

4. Confirm commitment

"How quickly will the Unconscious Mind begin? And how quickly will it finish, knowing this is for your highest good?"

Why This Works

By pinning the healing process to a specific timeframe, you create a sense of urgency and focus for the Unconscious Mind. Left unchecked, the Unconscious might delay or take the 'path of least resistance' to avoid change.

You can guide the Unconscious to act with purpose by reinforcing specific parameters that are:

- immediate (starting now),

- realistic (aligned with the body's natural rhythms)

- positive (connected to the client's outcome).

Overcoming Resistance to Timelines

Sometimes the client's Unconscious Mind may resist committing to a timeline. Follow these steps to handle it.

1. Reassure it

"It's perfectly fine if you'd like to organise the steps first — just as long as we know when you'll start and finish."

2. Introduce the path of least resistance

"Sometimes healing happens quickly because the body and mind naturally find the easiest and fastest way to complete the process."

3. Celebrate any movement forward

"Even if it begins slowly, every step your Unconscious Mind takes is moving you closer to the result."

Final Thoughts

Healing has natural timeframes — learn basic body processes, such as the stomach lining renewing over several days, liver tissue regenerating over time, and many other natural cycles of repair and renewal.

The Unconscious Mind works best when directed clearly — ask it to commit to when the process starts and when it will finish.

Use immediacy ('start now'), specificity ('finish in five days') and positivity ('feel calm and energised') to frame the change.

These tools empower you so you can confidently guide your client's Unconscious Mind to achieve rapid, effective results in a way that feels natural and aligned with their body's rhythm. By mastering this, you set your clients up for success and give them a profound experience of their ability to heal and change.

By elaborating on each step of the General Hypnosis Paradigm, you give yourself a clear and structured approach to Ericksonian interventions. Each step works harmoniously with the Unconscious Mind, creating space for discovery, acceptance, and powerful transformation.

Our trainings teach you to trust the process, follow your client's responses and adapt these steps naturally. With practice, you'll master this flexible framework to guide clients toward the deep and lasting change they desire.

Chapter 21:

The Pendulum and Other Ideomotor Signals

The General Hypnosis Paradigm introduced in the previous chapter outlined a clear and practical structure for communicating directly with the Unconscious Mind. One of the most powerful tools to facilitate that communication — especially in the early stages of trance work — is the pendulum.

The pendulum provides a gentle yet highly effective way to establish a dialogue with the Unconscious Mind, particularly when deeper trance phenomena have not yet emerged, or when the client is not quite ready to consciously explore the root cause of an issue. Using the pendulum allows you to receive clear unconscious signals that guide the session, build confidence and help the client feel reassured and supported throughout the process.

What is the Pendulum?

A pendulum is a simple yet remarkable biofeedback device. It works by amplifying tiny, unconscious muscle movements generated by the client's Unconscious Mind. These subtle movements create a visible response: the pendulum swings, circles or moves directionally in ways that can be easily interpreted. The pendulum bridges the gap between the Conscious and Unconscious Mind, offering an easy, non-confrontational way for the Unconscious to express itself directly and naturally.

Although commonly referred to simply as 'the pendulum' in modern hypnosis practice, it is historically known as Chevreul's Pendulum, named after

Michel Eugène Chevreul, the 19th-century French scientist who first investigated the phenomenon. Chevreul demonstrated that the pendulum's movements were not supernatural but instead arose from unconscious micro-movements of the muscles — movements directed by thought, attention and unconscious processes. Today, hypnotherapists use this natural ideomotor response to open up lines of communication with the Unconscious Mind, accessing insights, establishing yes/no signals, and gently guiding the internal processes necessary for deep transformation.

When to Use a Pendulum

The pendulum can be used when:

- a client struggles to visualise or concentrate

- a client has resistance to entering a formal trance state

- a gentle approach is needed to address a presenting issue without diving into its root cause

- you need a powerful convincer for clients who doubt their connection to the Unconscious Mind.

It can also be a useful complement to formal trance work. Many clients are amazed to see the pendulum responding, which builds their confidence in their ability to create change.

Case Study: Releasing Sleep Disturbance

Here is a powerful example of using the pendulum in a session.

Background: A woman came to see my mentor three days after experiencing a brutal mugging. She had been waking up screaming every night since the attack. While she wasn't ready to confront the traumatic memory, she desperately wanted relief and to sleep through the night.

Session: He introduced the pendulum to create communication with her Unconscious Mind.

1. He began with, *"Can I have a signal for 'yes'?"* and waited for the pendulum to swing in a clear direction.

2. He then asked, *"And now a signal for 'no'?"* and confirmed the response.

3. He asked, *"Does your Unconscious Mind know what to do to help you sleep soundly through the night?"*

The pendulum signalled *'yes'*.

4. *"Is it possible to release the negative emotions needed to achieve that?"* Again, the pendulum signalled 'yes'.

5. *"Is it okay to release those emotions now?"* The pendulum signalled, "no".

At this point, he explored further:

- *"Would you like to start in 12 hours?"* (Yes.)

- *"How quickly will you finish? Would you like to complete this in 36 hours?"* (Yes.)

Outcome: That night, the woman woke up screaming again, but the next night — and every night afterward — she slept soundly through the night. Her Unconscious Mind took the time it needed to begin releasing the emotions safely and gently. This general intervention brought her relief, while allowing her to seek help for the root cause when ready.

Setting Up the Pendulum Position (and Using Arm Catalepsy)

Before you begin using the pendulum, it's important to set up the client's hand and arm comfortably and correctly.

- Ask the client to sit comfortably at a table or desk, resting their elbow firmly on the tabletop.

- Guide their forearm to an almost upright (vertical) position, so it is in the shape of a 'V'.

- Let their hand relax completely from the wrist, so the fingers dangle loosely and naturally.

As you move their hand and arm into place, you can gently induce arm catalepsy (also called waxy flexibility) — a natural light trance phenomenon. Here's the key: use very light, almost ambiguous, touch as you guide their hand.

Touch the client's wrist or hand so lightly that they can't quite tell the exact moment when your touch ends. Their Unconscious Mind will focus on the sensation of that barely-there touch, and while they are engaged with it, the arm will often stay suspended comfortably all by itself — without any conscious effort.

This method is based on Milton Erickson's sensory ambiguity technique used to turn attention inward, and it's a powerful way to create both physical stillness and Unconscious engagement right at the start. When you do this successfully:

- the arm feels effortlessly supported

- the client naturally slips into a light trance

- the pendulum becomes easier to use and responds more clearly to unconscious signalling.

By combining proper positioning with the gentle induction of arm catalepsy, you create the perfect foundation for using the pendulum with ease and success.

Here is the step-by-step process to use the pendulum with a client.

1. Setting up the pendulum

1. Use a pendulum with a finger clip for stability. If you don't have a finger clip pendulum, a ring with a weighted balanced object/ pendulum on a string or light chain will work. If this isn't possible, holding the pendulum string/light chain between thumb and forefinger is acceptable, but the least preferred option.

2. Have the client sit at a table or desk. Ask them to rest their elbow on the surface, or guide them and induce arm catalepsy while positioning their arm, so their forearm is vertical (in the shape of a 'V') and their hand is relaxed and hanging from the wrist.

3. Attach the pendulum to their finger and ensure it can swing freely.

2. Elicit signals from the Unconscious Mind

Begin by introducing the pendulum and explaining its role: *"Your Unconscious Mind will use tiny muscle movements to communicate through the pendulum. Let's set up signals so we can easily understand each other."*

a. Getting a clear 'yes' signal from the Unconscious Mind

Once the pendulum is positioned correctly and the client's hand is relaxed, it's time to invite a response from the Unconscious Mind.

Start by saying something like: *"Let's invite your Unconscious Mind to give us a signal for 'Yes' — a signal that's easy for both of us to see. Sometimes the Unconscious Mind likes to create a 'Yes' signal by swinging the pendulum back and forth like this …"*

Demonstrate by holding the pendulum almost horizontal and gently letting it swing either front to back or side to side.

Then add: *"Other times, the Unconscious Mind might prefer to swing the pendulum a different way for 'Yes' — and that would be just as perfect."* (Show the pendulum swinging in a different direction, such as side to side if you first demonstrated front to back.)

This simple demonstration gives the client's Unconscious Mind a physical example — a feeling for what kind of movement is acceptable.

Now invite them to find their own signal by saying: *"Now, inside your mind, you can ask your Unconscious Mind to show us a clear signal for 'Yes.' Just repeat silently to yourself, 'Signal for Yes, Signal for Yes, Signal for Yes.' And just allow it to happen."*

Pause here and give plenty of time for the first movement to emerge. Sometimes it starts small — a tiny swing or a slight pull.

If the movement is very faint or hard to see, gently encourage the Unconscious Mind:

- *"That's good. And now, could your Unconscious Mind make that signal even stronger and easier for us to see? That's right … just allowing it to become more noticeable now."*

- *"Can you amplify that signal so it's very easy to see?"*

If you are using a pendulum chart (a simple guide showing directions for 'Yes' and 'No'), you can place it under the pendulum at this point and align it to the initial 'Yes' direction.

b. Ask for a 'No' signal

Once the 'Yes' signal has been established, then steady the pendulum and say: *"Dear Unconscious Mind, and now show me a signal for 'No'?"*

Key note: Specific language is important. If you ask the Unconscious Mind could you show me a signal for 'no', the Unconscious Mind could respond with yes (because YES it could). Be clear with your language.

c. Ask for a 'Not Ready' signal

This allows the Unconscious Mind to communicate when it is not ready to give an answer: *"Dear Unconscious Mind, and now give me a signal for 'Not Ready' meaning not consciously ready to know or 'I don't know' or 'Not Sure'."*

3. Begin the dialogue

Follow the General Hypnosis Paradigm from the previous chapter. Ask questions like:

- *"Does your Unconscious Mind know what to do to solve the problem?"*

- *"Is it possible to release what is necessary to resolve this now?"*

- *"Is it okay to begin this process now?"*

- *"How quickly will the process begin? How quickly will it finish?"*

4. Maintain rapport

As the pendulum swings, acknowledge the signals to deepen the client's comfort and trust: *"That's right. Thank you, Unconscious Mind, for communicating so clearly."*

5. Use the pendulum chart (optional)

Place a pendulum chart under the pendulum with clear markings for yes, no and not sure. This visual aid can make the process even clearer for the client.

Why the Pendulum Works

The pendulum operates on ideomotor signals — tiny, involuntary muscle movements influenced by the Unconscious Mind. This process allows clients to bypass their Conscious Mind and communicate directly with their deeper self.

It also serves as a powerful convincer. When clients see the pendulum move, it deepens their belief in the process and their ability to connect with their Unconscious Mind. This creates an ideal state for change work.

Other Ideomotor Signals

Ideomotor signalling is simply the Unconscious Mind expressing itself through small, automatic physical movements — a gentle way to create clear two-way communication during hypnosis.

Milton Erickson and Ernest Rossi taught that the best ideomotor responses often happen naturally, without force or heavy direction. They focused on simple, spontaneous movements like:

- a finger twitch

- a slight hand lift

- a head nod or small head shake.

Their approach was based on trusting the Unconscious Mind to choose its own easiest, most natural form of communication.

Since Erickson's time, additional methods have been developed by hypnotherapists and trainers to make ideomotor signalling even more accessible, especially when working with beginners or structured learning environments. These include:

- the Sticky Finger Test, which uses sensation to create unconscious responses

- The ABCDE Finger Signals, which allow for quick yes/no/multiple-choice communication.

These modern techniques honor Erickson's original spirit — inviting, never forcing — while offering more options to help clients and students find the clearest and most comfortable way to respond.

Whether using a pendulum, a hand movement or a shift in sensation, the core principle remains the same: the Unconscious Mind already knows how to communicate — our role is simply to notice and follow.

1. Sticky Finger Test (Sensory-Based Ideomotor Signal)

This is a simple method to elicit unconscious responses through a change in sensation.

How to do it:

- Ask the client to gently rub the tip of their index finger across a waxy or textured surface, such as a notebook cover or glossy piece of paper.

- Say: *"Dear Unconscious Mind give me a signal for 'Yes' — maybe a little extra stickiness, or a slight feeling of drag. Signal for Yes, Signal for Yes …"*

- Allow time for them to notice a difference.

- Then ask for a 'No' signal and notice the changes in feeling, drag or stickiness.

Why it works: Subtle changes in sensation often bypass conscious control, allowing unconscious responses to come through easily.

2. ABCDE Finger Signals (Multiple-Choice Ideomotor Signalling)

Perfect for when you want more than just a 'Yes' or 'No' response.

How to do it:

- Have the client rest their non-dominant hand on their lap (or overhanging on their knee) with fingers relaxed and loose.

- Label each finger: thumb = A; index finger = B; middle finger = C; ring finger = D; little finger = E.

- Invite the Unconscious Mind: *"you can allow one of the fingers to lift, twitch or move slightly to choose an answer."*

- Start by asking for a 'Yes' or 'No' practice signal, then move into multiple-choice questions as needed.

Tip: Movements may be very small at first — barely a twitch — so watch closely and affirm all attempts.

3. Head Nods and Head Shakes

Some clients prefer using larger body movements.

How to do it:

Invite the client's Unconscious Mind to create a tiny head nod for 'Yes' and a slight shake for 'No'.

Remind them that even the intention to move is enough for the signal to happen.

4. Hand Lift as Ideomotor Signal

This signal is another Ericksonian classic.

How to do it:

Invite the Unconscious Mind to gently lift a finger, a few fingers or even the entire hand.

It may start as a light floating feeling or an urge to move.

Hand lifts can also be used later for deeper trance phenomena, regression work or unconscious signalling during therapy.

Key Reminders for All Ideomotor Work:

- Invite, don't push.

- Allow any movement, however small. Tiny movements are perfect.

- Celebrate all responses as successes — even very small ones.

- Trust the Unconscious Mind's timing and methods.

Favourite Phrases to Use

- "You might notice it starting to happen now, all by itself…"

- "There's no need to rush — just allow the signal to emerge naturally."

- "Even the slightest feeling or urge is perfect."

Final Thoughts

The pendulum and other ideomotor tools are simple yet profound methods for working with the Unconscious Mind. They create a bridge of communication, allowing clients to move forward with clarity and trust. Whether used as part of a formal trance or as a standalone tool, they reinforce the transformative process that lies at the heart of our approach.

Using the Pendulum to Increase Metabolism

Hypnotherapists trained in advanced techniques learn how to unlock the potential of the Unconscious Mind to create lasting, transformative change. One of the fascinating applications explored in our Master Practitioner Hypnosis Training is how to use the pendulum to influence physiological processes, such as increasing metabolism.

The pendulum becomes more than just a communication tool; it evolves into a gateway for initiating profound physiological shifts.

How It Works

In this advanced technique, students learn to engage the Unconscious Mind in a focused dialogue to influence the body's metabolic processes. The process involves:

1. Setting the frame

During the session, the hypnotherapist explains to the client that the Unconscious Mind is the master regulator of all bodily functions, including metabolism. They set the intent that the pendulum will facilitate communication with the Unconscious Mind to support positive metabolic change.

2. Eliciting pendulum signals

Using the pendulum chart, students guide the client in identifying clear 'yes', 'no' and 'not yet' signals. This ensures smooth and reliable communication throughout the process.

3. Asking targeted questions

The hypnotherapist then asks questions, such as:

- "Does your Unconscious Mind know how to increase your metabolism to a healthy and optimal rate?"

- "Is it possible to speed up your metabolism while maintaining balance in your overall health?"

- "Is it okay to start increasing your metabolism today?"

Each response from the pendulum strengthens the client's belief in their ability to influence their body's processes.

4. Giving direct suggestions

The Unconscious Mind is directed to regulate metabolism efficiently. For example:

- "Unconscious Mind, go ahead and optimise the metabolic processes, ensuring your body converts energy in the most efficient and healthy way possible."

- "How quickly would you like to start? Would you prefer to begin now, or within the next 12 hours?"

- "How long will it take to achieve the ideal safe and healthy metabolic state? Will it be a day? Two days? Or more gradual over a week?"

5. Providing feedback loops

The pendulum is used to confirm the Unconscious Mind's agreement to these suggestions and to refine the timeline for achieving results.

TIP : If you ever feel like the pendulum is "not moving", don't push. Treat it as information. Slow down, build safety, re-explain the process and start with gentle, uncomplicated questions. Starting small helps the Unconscious Mind feel safe, cooperative and ready to communicate.

Why This Matters:

By incorporating advanced pendulum techniques, such as increasing metabolism, students experience firsthand how powerful this tool can be in creating measurable physical changes. This bridges the gap between the mind and body, making these techniques highly applicable to weight management, energy optimisation and overall health enhancement.

During our Clinical Diploma of Hypnotherapy & NLP pathway, we dive deep into the interplay between hypnosis, physiology and the Unconscious Mind. Students will master not only pendulum techniques for influencing metabolism but also tools to regulate other processes, such as reducing inflammation, enhancing immunity, improving hormonal balance and so much more. Mastery of these skills can open up exciting possibilities for helping clients achieve transformational results!

Chapter 22:

Metaphors – The Art of Guiding Transformation

Metaphors are one of the most powerful tools in hypnosis, NLP and change work. They hold a unique ability to bypass the Conscious Mind's defenses and speak directly to the Unconscious Mind. In my experience, metaphors have the potential to create profound and lasting transformations in a way that feels natural, effortless and even enjoyable.

Whether you are new to hypnosis or an experienced trainer, understanding and utilising metaphors can elevate your practice and provide meaningful insights to your clients. This chapter is designed to help anyone — students, trainers or practitioners — grasp the concept of metaphors and learn how to use them effectively in any change work.

Why Metaphors Are Essential in Hypnosis

Earlier in this book, we explored the hypnotic language patterns of the Milton Model — a way of using permissive, indirect language to create trance naturally. One of the key principles you learned is this: ambiguity creates trance.

Milton Erickson, the father of modern hypnotherapy, discovered over his lifetime that he could lead a person into a deep, receptive trance state simply by telling stories — stories that captured the curiosity of the Unconscious Mind. These stories are called metaphors.

Wouldn't it be wonderful to:

- captivate your client with a story that keeps them intrigued?

- craft a narrative that opens their mind to new possibilities and solutions?

- help clients shift from feeling stuck to accessing powerful resources for change?

Metaphors are tools for transformation. They allow you to:

- Bypass conscious resistance: instead of addressing the problem head-on, a metaphor works indirectly, preventing the Conscious Mind from interfering.

- Induce trance naturally: a well-told metaphor can subtly guide your client into a state of focused attention, where deeper change is possible.

- Loosen the grip of problems: metaphors can unravel limiting beliefs and rigid patterns of thinking, sometimes resolving the issue without direct intervention.

- Engage the Unconscious Mind: the Unconscious Mind loves stories. Through metaphors, it can access new perspectives and resources to create solutions.

The Power of Telling Stories

Erickson discovered that when he told a story without completing it, the story would cause the Unconscious Mind to lean in, searching for meaning and resolution. This 'open loop' created a state of focus and curiosity — the ideal mindset for therapeutic change.

A metaphor is a story told with intention. Unlike casual storytelling, a therapeutic metaphor has a purpose: to create a connection between the client's problem and a possible resolution. This connection, however, remains outside their conscious awareness.

Key Principles of Metaphors

- Purposeful storytelling: every element of the metaphor — its characters, setting and journey — is designed to parallel the client's experience in some way.

- Ambiguity: the story's connection to the client's problem should remain subtle, so the Conscious Mind doesn't interfere.

- Pacing and leading:

  ○ Pace: start by describing the client's current state indirectly through the metaphor.

  ○ Lead: gradually guide the story toward the resources and resolution the client needs.

- Universal or personalised: while you can use general themes (e.g. a lighthouse guiding ship), tailoring the story to the client's interests, hobbies and experiences makes it even more effective.

How to Craft a Transformative Metaphor

Step 1: Understand the client's problem

Before writing your metaphor, analyse the client's current state:

- How to they "do" their problem? (What are the patterns, beliefs or behaviours keeping them stuck?)

- What resources or steps could help them? (Consider what they might need to see, hear or feel to move forward.)

Remember, the story is designed to help move them from their present state/situation to their desired state/situation.

Step 2: Choose a theme

Select a subject that resonates with the client. This could be something from their personal interests or hobbies, or a neutral topic like nature, art or teamwork. Some examples include:

- Gardening: a seed struggling to grow until it finds the right soil

- Music: learning a new piece that feels impossible at first but becomes effortless with practice

- The ocean: waves crashing against rocks but finding their way back to the shore

- Lighthouses: A beacon guiding ships safely through a storm.

Step 3: Design the journey

Create a story where the main character experiences a challenge similar to the client's problem. Ensure that the character accesses resources, learns new perspectives or takes steps that lead to resolution.

Step 4: Write open-loop metaphors

In hypnotherapy, we often use open loops, where stories are started but left incomplete. This excites the Unconscious Mind's curiosity and draws the client into a deeper state of focus.

1. Start with the first metaphor: open the first story, then move to the second, third, fourth and then fifth. Leave each story incomplete at a moment of suspense or curiosity. (In practice, 3 – 5 metaphors seems to be ideal. Beyond 12, impact can dilute rather than deepen.)

2. Do the Change Work: once the client is deeply engaged, proceed with your therapeutic intervention.

3. Close the loops: after the intervention, finish the stories in reverse order, starting with the fifth, then the fourth, the third, the second and, finally, finish the first metaphor. This elegantly brings the client out of trance while reinforcing the change work.

Step 5: Practise and refine

Practise telling your metaphors to a colleague or friend. Pay attention to their reactions and adjust your pacing, tone and breaks to maximise the impact.

Let's do the deep dive and explore some open-loop metaphors to experience how it all comes together.

Open Loop 1: The Gardener's Journal

It's often said that true mastery of anything doesn't happen overnight ... It grows. Quietly. Steadily. In ways not always visible at first glance.

There once was a gardener ... who loved her land more than words could say. Each morning, before the world fully woke, she would walk barefoot along narrow garden paths ... pausing to notice how certain leaves tilted ever so slightly toward the dawn ... while others tucked themselves shyly into shade.

She carried with her a journal so thick it barely fit in her hands ... page after page ... notes about the texture of the earth ... the scent just before a summer storm ... the way one petal curled tighter than another. It was as if every detail demanded to be captured ... recorded ... preserved.

Yet as the seasons turned ... and turned again ... something curious began to happen. The journal grew thinner. One hundred pages became fifty. Fifty became thirty, then 29, 28, 27, 26, 25 ... Twenty-five became twenty, then 19, 18, 17, 16, 15, 14, 13, 12, 11 then ten became five. Then three. Then two. Then one.

Until eventually ... she walked with empty hands ... yet understood the garden more deeply than ever before.

And it was on one of those misty mornings ... just as a soft wind stirred the first golden leaves of autumn ...that something entirely unexpected appeared at the edge of her familiar path ...

(Leave open — no conclusions — move directly to Open Loop 2.)

Open Loop 2: The Locked Library

If there were a gift you could place gently into someone's hands ...the kind of gift that changes everything without needing to be unwrapped ... perhaps it would be the gift of curiosity. The deep, effortless kind ... that pulls you forward without even thinking about it. The kind that leads you to places you didn't know you needed to find.

Tucked behind the winding halls of an old museum ... beyond the rooms anyone visits ... there was a door. No signs. No explanations. Just the heavy hum of something waiting ... behind thick wood worn smooth by time and longing.

The townspeople never spoke of it openly ... but now and then, if you listened closely between conversations ... you might hear a whisper ... that behind that door ... were maps to places uncharted ... letters never delivered ... diaries written in languages that no longer exist.

And on certain afternoons, if you pressed your palm lightly against the door ... you could almost feel it ... a faint stirring ... like breath behind old stone ... or the delicate tremor of pages aching to be read.

There was a boy once ... or maybe he was something more than just a boy ... who wandered these halls when no one was watching. And somehow — no one knows quite how — he found a key.

Or perhaps ... the key found him.

It was small, unremarkable, almost easy to overlook. But when he held it ... there was a pull ... a knowing that had no words.

And when, at last, he placed the key into the lock ... there was a sound. A soft click. And then ... something began to move on the other side.

But what he discovered ... what waited beyond that threshold ... was nothing anyone could have expected.

(Leave open ... move to next open loop.)

Open Loop 3: The Musician and the Secret Code

There's a story I heard once ... about a young musician ... a girl who dreamed, not just of playing the violin, but of mastering it in a way that few ever could. She wasn't satisfied with playing the notes correctly ... she wasn't interested in applause ... or technique alone. She was searching for something deeper ... something hidden ... something that lived underneath the music itself.

Her teacher — an old man with kind eyes and a voice like velvet — once leaned in close and whispered: "If you really want to master this ... listen not just to the notes ... but to the spaces between them."

At first, she didn't understand. She practised scales until her fingers ached. She memorised every fingering, every tempo marking, every dynamic change. And yet ... the music still felt stiff ... mechanical ... flat. It was as if she were colouring inside the lines ... without ever seeing the picture.

Then one golden afternoon ... as the light poured through her window like liquid honey ... something shifted.

She set aside the sheet music ... closed her eyes ... and just listened.

At first, there was only silence ... then ... a single note. Rising ... falling ... vanishing into stillness.

And somewhere ... far beyond the notes ... in the pauses no one ever taught her to hear ... she noticed it. A presence. A pulse. A kind of breathing hidden within the music itself.

It was faint at first — a feeling more than a sound — as if the violin had always been speaking, but only now had she become quiet enough to listen.

And what she heard ... what she began to understand ... was not something that could be explained with words ... or captured in notes on a page. It was something that had to be felt ... sensed ... carried silently within.

Only ... what she heard ... was not meant for everyone to understand. Not at first.

(Leave open ... move to next open loop.)

Open Loop 4: The Salt Water Inlet

Along the southern edge of the peninsula, where the land breathes into the sea, there is an inlet so still that even the clouds seem to pause above it.

Here, the brackish waters — neither entirely of the ocean nor entirely of the land — stretch out like a silver mirror, rippling only with the softest sigh of the tide.

Locals speak of it in hushed voices, as though mentioning it too loudly might disturb the delicate spell woven there. They say that the inlet moves to a rhythm older than memory ... a slow, timeless dance of water and sky ... where the light changes minute by minute, yet somehow remains eternal.

Birds glide silently overhead — pelicans, black swans, Cape Barren geese, osprey — drifting so effortlessly it seems the very air carries them without thought. Every now and then, a quiet ripple betrays the movement of life beneath the surface — unseen but always present.

There was a man who came to that place. He had grown weary — not just in his body, but in something deeper. The kind of tiredness no sleep could cure, and no remedy could reach.

He had heard whispers of the inlet ... how people who visited often left with lighter steps and softer faces. And one morning, without really planning to, he found his way there.

He carried no expectations. No demands. Only a quiet hope that maybe ... just maybe ... being near something so ancient might remind him of something he had forgotten.

He sat near that inlet, drinking in its beauty and admiring the reflections. The breeze brushed against his skin like the touch of something remembering him.

He watched the light flicker across the water ... gold ... silver ... deep blue ... each colour shifting without hurry, without struggle. He listened to the gentle lapping at the water's edge — the inlet breathing, living, without needing to prove anything at all.

Minutes ... maybe hours ... passed without measure.

And somewhere between the ebb and flow of the tide, between the shifting reflections and the stillness beneath, something inside him ... softened. Shifted. Rearranged itself in a way he could not explain.

Was it the inlet itself that did this? The touch of the breeze? The silent acceptance of the water, reflecting everything without judgement?

Or was it something else entirely ... something waiting deep within him all along ... just waiting for the right place, the right moment, to awaken?

(Leave open ... move to next open loop.)

Open Loop 5: The Factory of Silent Signals

It's said that once, in a noisy factory, a young observer — not unlike Erickson himself — noticed something remarkable.

The factory was enormous ... its walls alive with the clanging of metal, the ticking of countless clocks being assembled, the steady hum and whirr of machines that seemed never to sleep.

At first glance, it was pure chaos. Workers weaving among conveyor belts ... crates stacked high ... parts scattered like confetti across long wooden benches. And the noise ... so thick and constant it wrapped itself around every movement, muffling even the loudest shout.

And yet ... in the heart of that noise ... something almost magical was happening.

The workers moved with effortless precision. Not a word spoken. Just a glance ... a tilt of the head ... a small shift of the shoulders ... a lift of an eyebrow almost too subtle to catch.

Entire sequences of action were triggered by these tiny cues. Gears fitted into gears. Clocks came to life. Movements cascaded ... perfectly ... silently ... as though some invisible thread connected them all.

And standing there, at the edge of that rhythmic, unseen dance, the young observer felt a sensation he couldn't quite name ... as if he were on the verge of understanding something he had always known ... but somehow forgotten.

And just as he leaned in closer ... drawn toward the delicate current of silent messages weaving through the noise ... something happened that changed the way he would listen forever ...

(Leave open.)

Suggestion/Therapy/Intervention Section

[Insert your suggestion, therapy or intervention work immediately after the last open loop — in this case, it is the Factory of Silent Signals — before you start closing the loops.]

This is my suggestion for you:

And as you continue to listen now ...perhaps even without realising it consciously ... you might begin to notice a very real and natural sense of confidence starting to grow inside you.

Because your Unconscious Mind already knows so much more than you think it does ... doesn't it? It knows how to learn easily ... naturally ... the way a river knows how to find the sea. It's not something you have to force. It's simply something you allow. Allow it now.

And maybe you can begin to imagine ... just how effortless it can be to grow these skills ... to discover, day by day, that the words you need ... the awareness you seek ... the understandings you desire ... are already there, ready to emerge, like seeds awakening after the rain.

You might find yourself becoming more and more curious ... about the ways your hands can move just a little differently ... the way your voice can change its tone just a little more smoothly ... the way you can listen — really listen — to the spaces between the words, to the subtle messages that were always there, just waiting for you to notice.

And the more you relax into this learning ... the more you can trust that every session you have, every practice you do, every story you tell ... is simply another step along a path that you are already walking so beautifully well.

Because you already have within you everything you need to become the hypnotist you are meant to be. And the Unconscious Mind ... your greatest ally ... is always ready to guide you ... support you ... and lead you exactly where you need to go.

Now ... as you continue to absorb these realisations ... and allow this new confidence to weave itself through every part of who you are becoming ... soon it will be time to return ... to complete the stories we began ... and to bring with you everything you have discovered.

Closing the Loops (in Reverse Order)

Close Loop 5: The Factory of Silent Signals

And long after the noise of the factory had faded from his ears ... the young observer would remember that precise moment — the one where he had leaned in ... listening beyond the clang and rattle, into something quieter, finer, more delicate than sound itself.

It wasn't a word, or a gesture or even a look that taught him.

It was a realisation — that beneath every conversation, every movement, every silence, there are currents ... invisible threads that people send out, without even knowing they do.

And from that day forward, he listened differently.

He noticed the hesitation before a sentence was spoken ... the shift in breathing when a feeling stirred ... the way the energy in a room could tilt — almost imperceptibly — when truth was near.

He had learned that real communication ... the kind that matters most ... often arrives before the words ever catch up.

And with that understanding, he found he could hear what most others missed entirely — the silent 'songs' people carried within them, waiting for someone ... finally ... to listen.

Close Loop 4: The Salt Water Inlet

In the weeks that followed his time at the inlet, the man noticed changes he could not fully name.

The weight he had carried for so long no longer pressed heavily on his chest. His steps felt lighter, somehow ... more certain. And though he still faced the same world ... he saw it now as if through a clearer lens — softer around the edges, more forgiving, more alive.

He returned to the inlet from time to time, not to seek answers, but simply to sit ... to listen ... to learn.

And each time he did, the tide would meet him as it always had — rising and falling ... offering no demands, making no judgements ... only reflecting back whatever he brought with him.

He never did explain to anyone exactly what had changed. Some things, he realised, are not meant to be explained.

They are meant to be experienced. Felt. Trusted.

Like the tide. Like the inlet. Like the deep, natural healing that happens when the mind grows quiet ... and simply remembers how to listen.

And so, the inlet remained a place of quiet refuge — a reminder that within stillness, profound transformation can unfold.

Close Loop 3: The Musician and the Secret Code

And in the years that followed ... as the young musician played on grand stages and in small, dark rooms alike ... those who listened often found themselves pausing ... caught in a moment between breaths ... where the air itself seemed to hum with something unspeakable.

Few could explain it. Many never even noticed it consciously. But something inside them responded — to the spaces ... to the silences ... to the music beneath the music.

And though she never spoke of it openly ... the musician knew ... that what she had found that day — hidden between the notes — was not something she could teach directly. It was something that others would have to discover for themselves ... in their own way ... in their own time ... in the quiet spaces where real understanding waits.

Close Loop 2: The Locked Library

And when the boy — or whatever he truly was — turned the key in the heavy door ... the hinges gave a soft groan, as if waking from a long and ancient sleep.

The door swung open, not quickly, but with a kind of patience ... revealing a room that seemed far larger on the inside than it could have been from without.

Shelves spiraled upward into shadow ... books and scrolls that shimmered as if breathing softly ... maps where ink shifted and shimmered when looked at sideways.

But what he discovered wasn't just words ... or pages ... it was something far more elusive.

It was the feeling ... of stepping into a place that had been waiting for him all along ... a place where every question had already been asked ... and every answer was simply waiting for the right moment to be found.

And as he stepped forward, beyond the threshold, into that place of wonder ... he understood — without needing to name it — that some doors don't stay locked forever. They simply wait ... until curiosity turns the key.

Close Loop 1: The Gardener's Journal

And on that misty autumn morning, as the gardener walked beyond the edges of her familiar paths, she discovered a single new seedling growing where no seed had ever been planted.

No journal could have predicted it. No plan had accounted for it. It had simply appeared ... because the conditions were right. Because nature — like growth, like learning — unfolds best when we stop trying to control it ... and simply nurture what is already happening.

And from that day forward, she walked her garden with a lighter step ... trusting more ... worrying less ... knowing that real mastery was something that grew all on its own ... in its own time ... in its own perfect way.

Why Open Loops Work

Leaving a story incomplete excites the Unconscious Mind's natural drive for resolution. The mind stays open, searching, curious — and during this period, deeper work can happen.

Later, once the therapeutic change has been made, you close the loops by finishing the stories, providing satisfaction and reinforcing the change.

You'll notice that when the loops are closed, the client naturally feels a sense of completion — often feeling refreshed, lighter, or simply "different".

Tips for Effective Metaphors

- Make it descriptive: use vivid, descriptive language to help the client see, hear and feel the story's journey.

- Break at key moments: leave each story unfinished just before a pivotal event, keeping the client curious. Think cliffhanger!

- Keep it ambiguous: avoid explicitly connecting the metaphor to the client's issue. Let their Unconscious Mind make the connection.

- Test and observe: practise with real clients and observe their responses. Refine your metaphors based on their reactions.

Exercises for Students

Write Five Metaphors:

- Think of a specific client and their presenting problem.

- Choose five themes and craft stories that are two minutes each.

- Imagine the effect each story will have on the client.

Practise Open Loops:

- Rehearse telling your metaphors with a partner.

- Break each story at a suspenseful moment, then move to the next.

Observe and Adjust:

- Notice where your partner becomes engaged or loses focus.

- Adjust your tone, pacing and breaks to optimise their experience.

Metaphors as Your Superpower

Metaphors are more than just stories; they are bridges to transformation. With practice, you can:

- inspire curiosity and engagement

- help clients access resources they didn't realise they had

- guide them toward profound and lasting change.

As you refine your skill in creating and delivering metaphors, remember that every story has the potential to change a life. So, take your time, let your creativity flow and enjoy the process of crafting metaphors that make a difference.

Chapter 23:

The Law of Cause and Effect in Hypnosis

Where True Change Begins

W "Every action has a consequence. Every thought has an effect. Every choice creates a result."

In the universe — and in life — very little happens by accident. There is a natural law that governs the way everything unfolds. It's called the Law of Cause and Effect, and it is one of the most powerful guiding principles you'll ever understand as a hypnotherapist.

This chapter will help you — and your clients — step into full empowerment by understanding the difference between living at Cause and being stuck at Effect.

What Is the Law of Cause and Effect?

The Law of Cause and Effect says: For every effect, there is a specific cause. And for every cause, there is an inevitable effect.

It's how the world works.

You plant a seed (cause) and a plant grows (effect). You speak kindly to someone (cause) and they smile (effect). You neglect your health (cause) and eventually feel run down (effect).

The law works whether you believe in it or not. It's as consistent as gravity.

The same is true for your thoughts, emotions and behaviours. You reap the effects of the internal and external causes you set in motion.

In Hypnosis: The Shift From Reaction to Creation

People are not actually describing a lack of desire when they say something like:

- "I want to stop smoking, but I just can't."

- "I know I should feel confident, but I freeze."

- "I'm trying to move forward, but life keeps getting in the way."

They're describing being at effect — caught in the emotional and behavioural consequences of earlier, often unconscious, causes.

Here's what we help them do instead:

- uncover the original cause

- interrupt the unconscious pattern

- replace it with an intentional, empowering cause — so the effect naturally changes.

Because trying to change the effect (like anxiety, procrastination, smoking) without addressing the cause (the internal program driving it) is like repainting a leaking wall instead of fixing the pipe behind it.

Cause vs Effect in Everyday Life

Let's simplify this.

At Cause	At Effect
"I create my results."	"Things just happen to me."
"I'll find a solution."	"There's nothing I can do."
"I am responsible for how I feel."	"They made me feel this way."

Being at cause doesn't mean you blame yourself. It means you take your power back.

You realise: "If I created this unconsciously … I can change it consciously."

That's empowerment. That's healing. That's the work of a skilled hypnotherapist.

Above the Line vs Below the Line Thinking

This concept is also explained using the metaphor of living above or below the line.

- Above the Line: ownership, accountability, responsibility

- Below the line: blame, excuse, denial

Above the line = empowerment.

Below the line = entrapment.

Just observe how someone talks and behaves, and you'll instantly hear where they are.

- "I've tried everything, but nothing works…" → below the line

- "I'll keep refining my approach until I get the result." → above the line

Are You an OAR or in BED?

Let's use a simple metaphor to lock this in: Are you holding an OAR (steering your boat), or lying in BED (drifting and stuck)?

OAR (Above the Line)	BED (Below the Line)
Ownership	Blame
Accountability	Excuses
Responsibility	Denial

An OAR floats. A BED sinks. When you hold the OAR, you steer your direction. When you lie in BED, you hope the current will somehow carry you where you want to go.

Clients Need to Be at Cause to Change

In hypnotherapy, our role is to gently move clients from effect to cause.

At effect, they might say:

- "My anxiety is because of my childhood."

- "I can't lose weight because I'm always stressed."

- "I sabotage relationships — it's just how I am."

They're looking for external forces to change, but true change happens inside-out.

At cause, they start saying:

- "My past shaped me, but I can choose how I respond now."

- "I'm learning how to manage stress in healthy ways."

- "I'm ready to create a different future."

This shift is transformational. Hypnosis is the bridge that helps them make it.

Cause vs Effect in You as a Practitioner

You'll notice the same patterns in yourself.

When a client doesn't respond to an induction, do you say: *"This isn't working — they must not be suggestible."* (effect)

Or do you say: *"What can I adjust in my approach to support them better?"* (cause)

When you live at cause, you become more flexible, resilient and powerful in your practice.

Why This Relates to the Unconscious Mind

Much of what your clients struggle with isn't conscious. It's deeply patterned.

You could say that the effect they're experiencing now (e.g. anxiety, fear, self-sabotage) is the result of an unconscious cause planted long ago.

Your job isn't to talk them into feeling better. It's to guide their Unconscious to release the old pattern and replace it with a new cause — one that generates healing, freedom and confidence.

This is why hypnosis works: it bypasses the Conscious Mind and speaks directly to the source.

Timeless Insight

"Between stimulus and response, there is a space. In that space lies our power to choose our response. In our response lies our growth and our freedom." [1]

That space is what you're opening up for your clients. It's the pause button before the automatic reaction. It's where cause can override effect.

"A client will not actualise behaviours that the hypnotist does not believe are true or possible."

This principle underscores why it is critical for hypnotherapists to have a strong belief in their client's ability to change and to maintain a positive, hopeful attitude during the therapy process.

So ask yourself:

- Do you believe change is possible — no matter how stuck the client feels?

- Are you at cause in your own thinking and practice?

---

1. Although this quote is frequently attributed to Viktor E. Frankl, the exact wording does not appear in Man's Search for Meaning or in any of Frankl's published works. The Viktor Frankl Institute reports that the source of the quote is unknown and notes that Stephen R. Covey encountered the statement in an anonymous library book and popularised it due to its alignment with Frankl's teachings. For an authentic Frankl reference expressing a similar idea, see: Viktor E. Frankl, Man's Search for Meaning, Beacon Press, Boston, 2006, p. 66 (original English ed. 1959; original German ed. 1946).

Say these affirmations to yourself — every time before working with a client:

- *"This is the world's greatest hypnotic subject."*

- *"They will give me continuous feedback so I can deliver the perfect induction and session."*

You are at cause. And because you believe in their success — they'll start believing too. This is not about forcing outcomes, it's about creating the conditions where change becomes possible.

Final Questions for Reflection

Ask yourself the following questions. Encourage your clients to do the same.

- Am I living at cause or effect?

- Am I choosing OAR or lying in BED?

- Am I reacting … or creating?

You are never stuck. There is always a new cause you can create. And when you create a new cause, the effect must follow.

That's the law.

Client Exercise: The Shift to Cause

Ask your client to write out one area of life where they feel stuck. Then ask them to answer the following questions:

- What am I currently blaming, excusing or denying?

- What would it sound like if I took full ownership?

- What new 'cause' could I put in place today?

This simple process can change their state — and their story — before they even close their eyes.

Chapter 24:

Conclusion — You Were Made for This

So here we are — at the end of this book, but very much at the beginning of your journey.

If you've come this far, you've already proven something powerful: you're curious, committed and capable of creating extraordinary change in your life and in the lives of others. And in case no one's told you this lately — that says a lot about who you are.

You've explored the foundational principles of hypnosis, debunked common myths and discovered that hypnosis is not some mysterious force done to people but rather a natural, learnable process that anyone (yes — anyone!) can experience and master. You've learned the keys to ethical practice, the structure of suggestions, the role of language and how to create deep, transformational rapport. You've even met giants like Dave Elman and Milton Erickson, whose legacy lives on every time a hypnotherapist helps a client finally feel peace where there was once pain.

But let's pause for a moment and ask an important question.

What does all this mean for you?

If you've, at the very least, completed the 3-day Modern Hypnosis training, it means you now know enough to start. To start practising. To start helping. To start believing that maybe, just maybe, you were made for this.

Because hypnosis isn't just about techniques. It's about people. It's about compassion. It's about waking up parts of the mind that have been asleep for far too long — and helping others remember who they really are.

At Successful Minds Institute, we believe in training world-class hypnotherapists who lead with heart and skill. So I want to leave you with three reminders as you move forward:

1. You don't need to be perfect to make a difference

You just need to be present. Be curious. Stay grounded. Every time you sit with a client, trust that your intention to serve is more important than getting every word "right". You'll grow as you go.

2. Keep practising — and keep playing

Practice doesn't make perfect; it makes permanent. The more you engage with the tools, the more naturally they'll become part of your language. Start small. Notice what works. And above all — keep your sense of play and wonder.

3. You're not alone

You're now part of a growing family of heart-centered professionals who are reshaping the future of healing. Whether you continue through our Clinical Diploma of Hypnotherapy & NLP, dive into Master Practitioner work, or simply help a friend feel better about themselves — that ripple matters. And we're right here with you.

One Last Thought

You may have noticed by now that hypnosis is about more than closing eyes or counting backward. It's about opening doors. Doors to possibility. Doors to potential. Doors to peace.

So as you close this book, take a deep breath ... and imagine the difference you could make, simply by believing in the power of the unconscious mind — and in your ability to work with it.

You were made for this.

Your mind is your greatest asset. And when used with skill, integrity, and the right training... It becomes one of the most powerful tools for transformation you will ever encounter.

With belief in your brilliance,

Cherry Farrow
Founder, Successful Minds Institute
Master Trainer of NLP & Hypnotherapy,
Trainer of Time Line Therapy™, Trainer of NLP Coaching
Creator of The Release System™ and The Quantum Healing Paradigm™

Professional Note: *The information in this book is designed to educate and inspire. It is not a substitute for professional medical or psychological care. Always work within your level of training and competence, recognise contraindications, and refer to appropriately qualified professionals where required. When used with integrity, care, and the right training, hypnosis can be one of the most powerful tools for transformation.*

Your Pathway Forward

By now, you understand something many people never truly realise. Hypnosis isn't something that is *done to you*. It's something you can learn, experience, and use to create real change, for yourself and for others.

While this book has given you the foundations, real mastery comes from doing.

In a live training environment, you will:

- Experience hypnosis yourself (and understand it from the inside out)

- Learn how to confidently guide others into trance

- Develop real, practical skills through structured practice

- Receive feedback, coaching, and refinement

- Understand when, why, and how to use each process effectively

- Build certainty in your ability to create lasting change

Successful Minds Institute, offers a clear certification pathway for those who feel called to go further.

You may choose to begin with our **MindFit™ Hypnosis Certification (3-Day Training)** — an immersive, hands-on experience where you learn the foundations of modern hypnosis and begin working with real processes immediately.

From there, you can continue into our **MindFit™ NLP & Hypnotherapy Practitioner and Master Practitioner Training**s, where you develop a deeper understanding of human behaviour, communication, and transformational change.

And if you feel a desire not only to practice but to lead, our **NLP Trainers Training and Hypnosis Trainers Training** provide the opportunity to teach, present, and build your own training, coaching or consulting business. Creating impact on a much larger scale.

Our signature **Clinical Diploma of Hypnotherapy & NLP** offers a comprehensive pathway into professional, clinical-level practice and is for those called to the highest level of skill and integration.

Your Next Step

If something inside you is saying, *"this is for me"*. Trust that!

Visit: *www.successfulminds.com.au* and connect with our fabulous team to find the right certification training and pathway for you.

www.ingramcontent.com/pod-product-compliance
Lightning Source LLC
Chambersburg PA
CBHW070950200526
45161CB00001BA/54